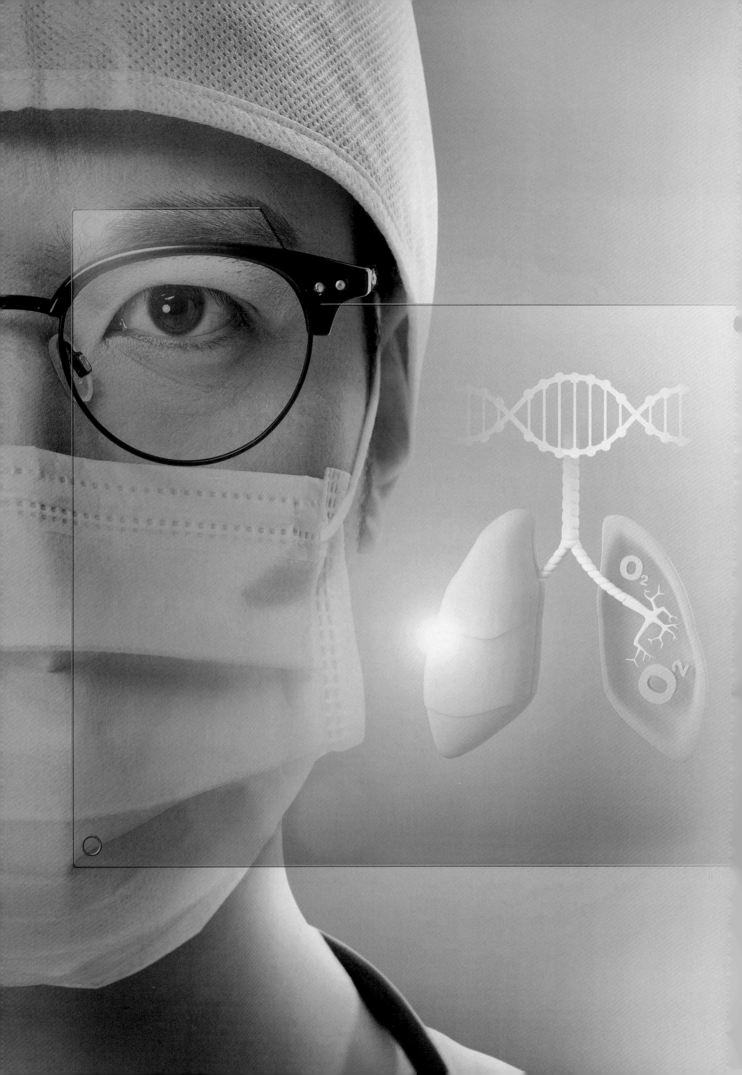

遏制结核
中国力量

Action in China to End TB

为了健康的呼吸

中国结核病防治纪实

For Breathing Healthily

Tuberculosis Control in China

中国疾病预防控制中心
中国健康教育中心
中国防痨协会
中国性病艾滋病防治协会　组织编写

Chinese Center for Disease Control and Prevention
Chinese Center for Health Education
Chinese Antituberculosis Association
Chinese Association of STD&AIDS Prevention and Control

人民卫生出版社
PEOPLE'S MEDICAL PUBLISHING HOUSE
·北　京·

要把人民健康放在优先发展战略地位，
努力全方位全周期保障人民健康。

——习近平

We should give top priority to people's health in our development strategy, and strive to ensure the delivery of comprehensive lifecycle health services for our people.

—President XI Jinping

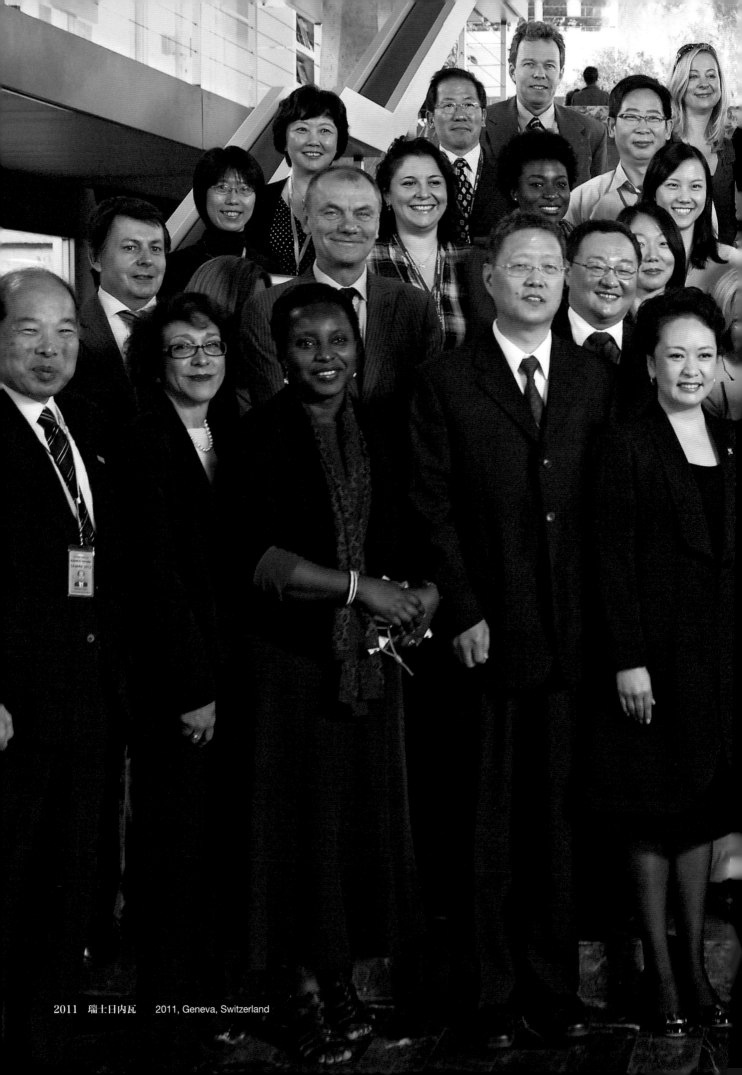

2011　瑞士日内瓦　　2011, Geneva, Switzerland

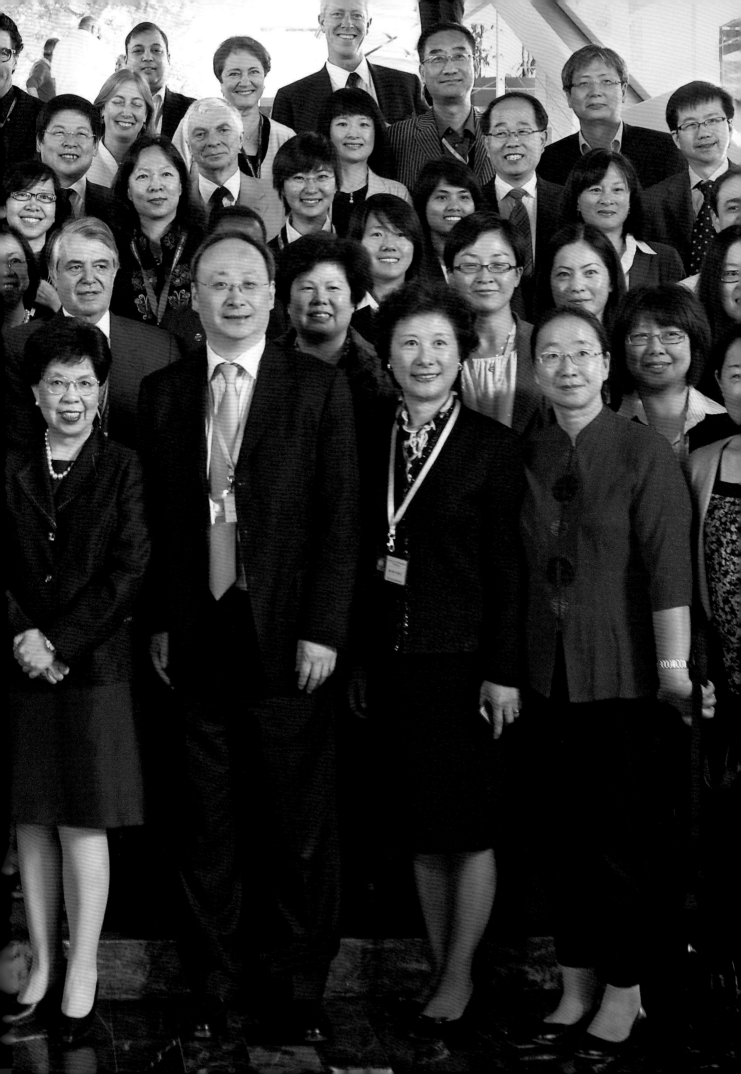

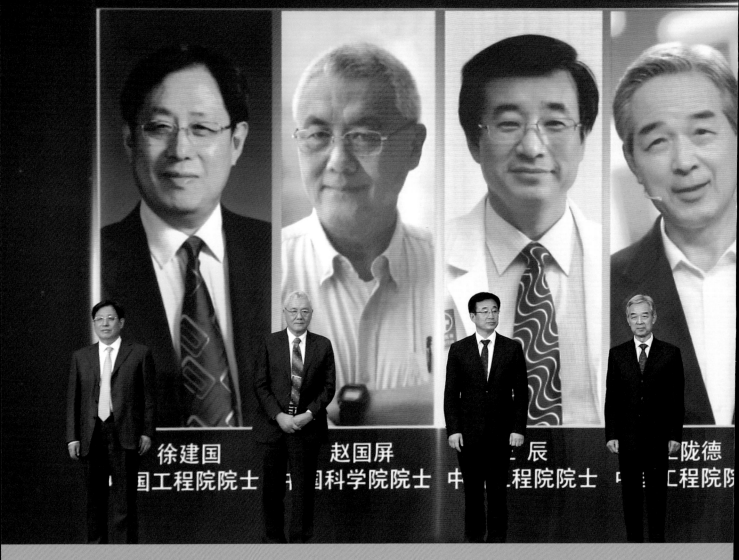

八位院士发起终结结核行动联合倡议
Eight academicians making a joint call for actions to end tuberculosis

高 福　中国科学院院士、病原微生物学、免疫学家
GAO Fu, Academician of the Chinese Academy of Sciences (CAS),
pathogenic microbiologist and immunologist

王陇德　中国工程院院士、公共卫生学家
WANG Longde, Academician of the Chinese Academy of Engineering (CAE)
and public health specialist

王 辰　中国工程院院士、呼吸病学家
WANG Chen, CAE academician and respiratory specialist

侯云德　中国工程院院士、病毒学、分子病毒学家
HOU Yunde, CAE academician, virologist and molecular virologist

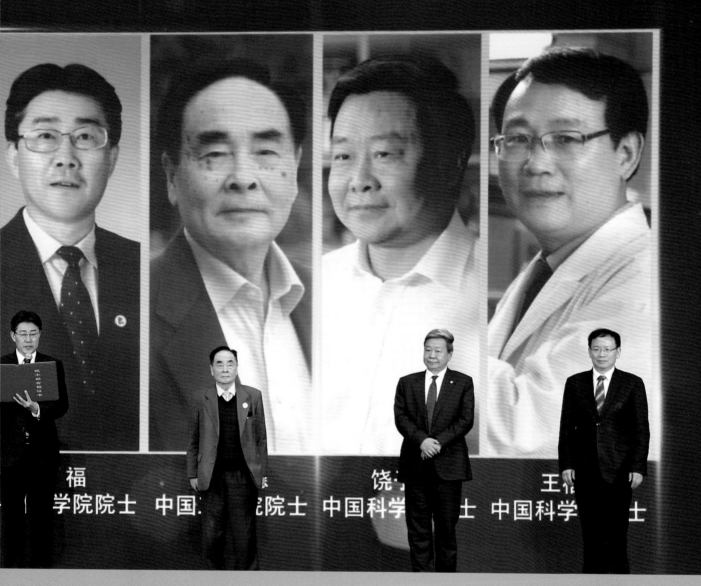

饶子和　中国科学院院士、分子生物物理与结构生物学家
RAO Zihe, CAS academician, molecular biophysicist and structural biologist

赵国屏　中国科学院院士、分子微生物学家
ZHAO Guoping, CAS academician and molecular microbiologist

徐建国　中国工程院院士、医学微生物学家
XU Jianguo, CAE academician and medical microbiologist

王福生　中国科学院院士、感染病学家
WANG Fusheng, CAS academician and specialist in infectious diseases

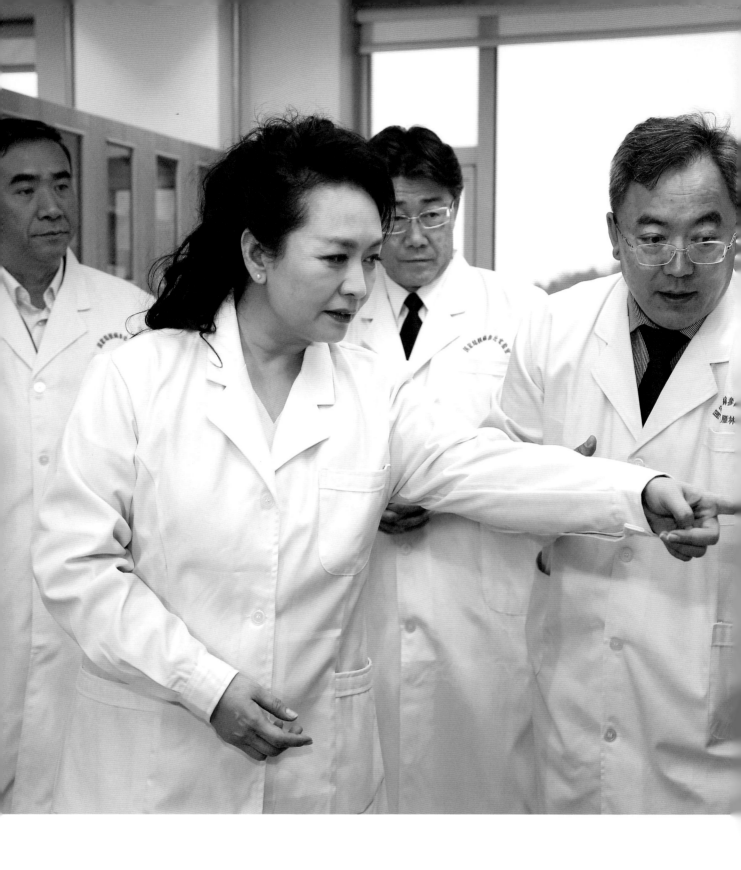

世界卫生组织结核病／艾滋病防治亲善大使彭丽媛考察结核病实验室
Peng Liyuan, WHO Goodwill Ambassador for TB and HIV/AIDS,
visited the tuberculosis laboratory

Over the years, under the strong leadership of the Party and government, and thanks to many years of commitment from health practitioners and hundreds of thousands of volunteers, China has achieved remarkable progress on tuberculosis control. Most notably, since the 2000s, China has successfully introduced and implemented DOTS strategy (Directly Observed Treatment, Short-course, the WHO tuberculosis treatment strategy) and developed a tuberculosis prevention and control service system with Chinese characteristics. Five years ahead of the schedule, China had achieved the United Nations Millennium Development Goals (MDGs) of halving the mortality and morbidity of tuberculosis, making a significant contribution to global tuberculosis control.

联合国可持续发展目标明确提出，到2030年实现全球终止结核病流行的目标。中国政府积极履行政治承诺，国家卫生健康委员会、国家发展改革委员会、教育部、科技部、民政部、财政部、国务院扶贫办和国家医保局联合制定了《遏制结核病行动计划（2019—2022年）》。各级卫生健康行政部门正在积极组织、认真落实健康中国行动计划，切实保护人民群众的身体健康，为中国乃至世界的结核病防治事业再创辉煌，为最终实现终止结核病流行的目标作出新的贡献！

The United Nations Sustainable Development Goals (SDGs) call for ending the epidemic of tuberculosis by 2030. The Chinese government has faithfully fulfilled its political commitments. The NHC, NDRC, MOE, MOST, MOCA, MOF and CPAD and NHSA jointly formulated the Tuberculosis Rollback Action Plan 2019-2022. Health commissions at all levels are actively mobilizing society-wide resources to earnestly implement major resolutions under the Healthy China strategy. This work includes continuing efforts, effectively safeguarding the health of the people, seeking greater success in fighting tuberculosis in China and beyond, and further contributing to the ultimate goal of ending tuberculosis!

盛世修史是中华民族的优良传统。在国家卫生健康委疾病预防控制局指导下，中国疾病预防控制中心、中国健康教育中心、中国防痨协会、中国性病艾滋病防治协会联合编写了《为了健康的呼吸——中国结核病防治纪实》，系统梳理了21世纪以来中国结核病防治服务体系的变迁，总结了防治工作取得的成绩，呈现了各地好的经验和做法，为社会各界了解和认识结核病提供参考借鉴。

To honor the Chinese tradition of documenting its proud history, under the guidance of Bureau of Disease Control, the National Health Commission, the China Center for Disease Control and Prevention, the China Center of Health Education, the Chinese Anti-Tuberculosis Association and the Chinese Association of STD and AIDS Prevention and control have jointly compiled this book, "For Breathing Healthily-Tuberculosis Control in China". The book systematically summarizes the changes of China's tuberculosis prevention and control services system since the 2000s, the achievements, and successful stories and best practices from all over China. This book can serve as a reference for public understanding of tuberculosis.

目录
Contents

第三章　体系建设　使命担当

Chapter 3　System Building of TB Control and Workforce with Mission in Mind

第四章　重点人群　精准施策

Chapter 4　Measures Targeted to Key Groups with the Right Strategies

第五章　智慧结控　技术创新
Chapter 5　Smart, Innovative and Forward-looking Approaches to TB Control

第六章　国际合作　发展共赢
Chapter 6　International Cooperation for Common Development

第七章　健康促进 全民参与

Chapter 7　Health Promotion and Universal Participation

第八章　公益大使 春风化雨

Chapter 8　Significant Impact of the Goodwill Ambassador

编后记

Postscript

第一章
政府承诺
消除结核

Chapter 1

Government Commitment to End Tuberculosis

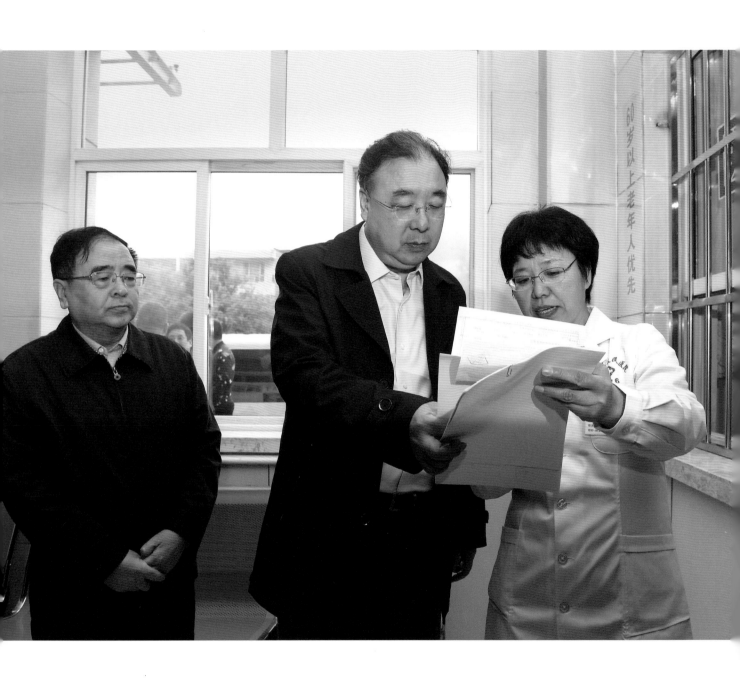

国家卫生健康委马晓伟主任考察基层卫生工作
Ma Xiaowei, director of the National Health Commission, inspected the primary health work
at the grass-roots level

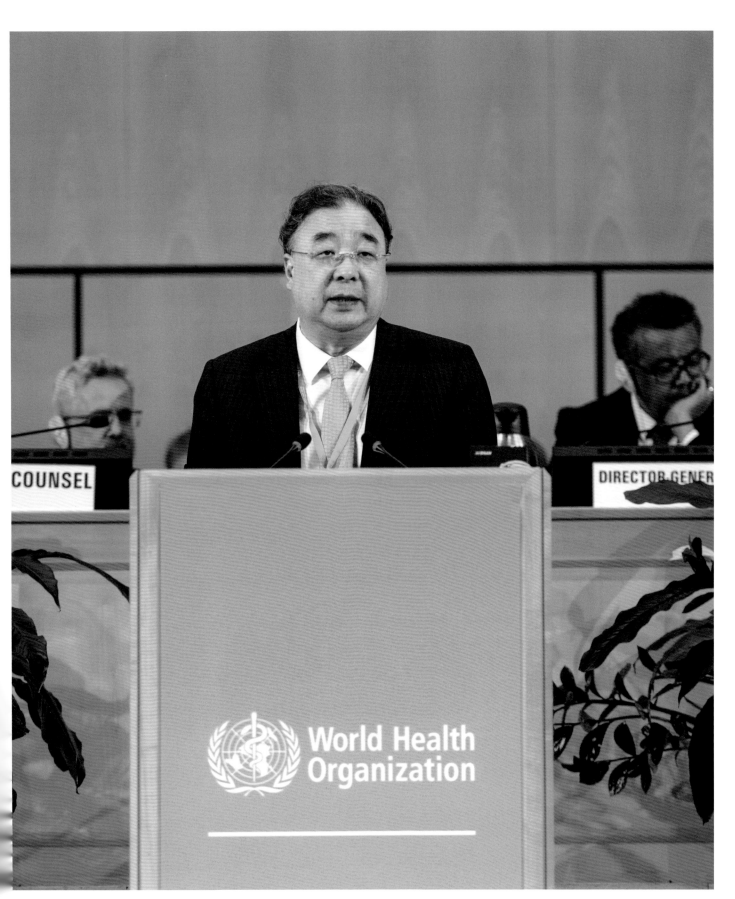

国家卫生健康委马晓伟主任出席第72届世界卫生大会
Ma Xiaowei, director of the National Health Commission, attended the 72nd World Health Assembly

党中央、国务院历来高度重视结核病防治工作，党的十八大以来，以习近平总书记为核心的党中央把防治结核病作为维护人民健康福祉的民生工程、民心工程，总书记在全国卫生与健康大会上做出全面部署，提出明确要求。回首21世纪以来中国结核病防治历程，我们始终坚持依法防治、科学防治、防治结合，防治工作取得了显著成绩，积累了宝贵经验。

The Communist Party of China's (CPC) Central Committee and the State Council have consistently attached great importance to the prevention and control of tuberculosis. Since the 18th National Congress of the Communist Party of China, the CPC Central Committee with General Secretary XI Jinping at its core has taken tuberculosis prevention and control as a livelihood project to maintain people's health and wellbeing and to boost morale of the people. President XI announced a comprehensive agenda and made clear-cut requirements during the National Health Conference. The experience of tuberculosis prevention and control in China since the 2000s suggests that China has adhered to the rule of law, respected science, and combined treatment with prevention and got remarkable achievements in the fight against tuberculosis with valuable experience accumulated for TB prevention and control.

始终坚持政府领导，不断健全政策法规。

Committed to government leadership and further improved policies and regulations.

成立了国务院防治重大疾病工作部际联席会议制度，将结核病作为重点疾病统一安排部署。颁布实施了《传染病防治法》和《结核病防治管理办法》，坚持依法防治，强化政府领导，明确政府、社会和个人的法律责任，确定了各级各类医疗卫生机构的职责和任务，保障了大众和结核病患者的健康权益。2001年以来，中国政府先后实施了三个结核病防治规划，分阶段确定防治目标、策略和措施。

An inter-agency joint taskforce for the prevention and control of major diseases was formalized under the State Council, and tuberculosis was identified as a priority for coordinated action. The *Law on the Prevention and Control of Infectious Diseases* and the *Administrative Measures for the Prevention and Control of Tuberculosis* were promulgated and enforced to stress prevention and control according to the law, strengthen government leadership, define the legal obligations of the relevant stakeholders (government, society and individuals), identify the responsibilities of medical and health institutions at all levels, and protect the rights for health of both the public and tuberculosis patients. Since 2001, the Chinese government has implemented three tuberculosis prevention and control programs and defined the objectives, strategies, and measures in stages.

始终坚持以人民为中心，不断完善防治策略。

Committed to people-centered care and constantly improved TB control strategies.

把维护人民健康权益放在首要位置，坚持"预防为主，防治结合"。全面落实三级预防策略，通过加强健康教育、提高全人群防护意识；对新生儿实施卡介苗接种，构筑免疫屏障；扩大筛查，及时发现传染源；完善治疗方案，规范患者管理，提高治愈率，切实保障人民健康。

People's rights to health was recognized as a primary priority. The strategy to fight tuberculosis was anchored in prevention and complemented by treatment. A three-tiered comprehensive prevention strategy was adopted. Health education campaigns were conducted to raise the awareness of tuberculosis and the measures taken to reduce the risks of contracting the disease. The neonatal BCG vaccination was administered to enhance immunity. Screening services were expanded to identify cases and prevent the spread of the disease in a timely manner. Treatment regimens were improved. Patient management was standardized. As a result of these efforts, the cure rate for tuberculosis has increased, which is a huge boon for people's health.

始终坚持防治服务体系建设，不断提高服务能力。

Committed to the service system construction for TB control and constantly and upgrade the service capacity.

2011年开始，中国逐步推进疾控机构、医疗机构和基层医疗卫生机构分工协作的"三位一体"结核病防治服务体系建设，提升结核病防治服务能力，确保预防、治疗、管理等各个环节间的无缝衔接。

Starting in 2011, China began to formalize the "3-in-1" TB prevention and control system with shared responsibilities and coordination among the CDCs, medical institutions, and primary healthcare organizations. The health system capabilities around tuberculosis prevention and control were also improved to ensure seamless integration among prevention, treatment, and patient management.

始终坚持多渠道筹资，不断加大保障力度。

Committed to diverse funding sources and increased protection.

中央财政设立结核病防治重大公共卫生专项，为患者筛查和一线抗结核药品提供补助，将结核病患者健康管理纳入国家基本公共卫生服务项目，由基层医疗卫生机构免费提供服药管理等服务。同时不断完善医疗保障政策，将抗结核药品纳入《国家基本药物目录》和医保目录，将耐多药肺结核诊疗纳入新农合和健康扶贫重大疾病保障范围，提高患者保障水平。

A significant and dedicated public health fund for tuberculosis prevention and control was set up in the central government budget to subsidize patient screening and first-line tuberculosis drugs. Health management for tuberculosis patients was integrated into the National Basic Public Health Service Program. Primary healthcare organizations were tasked to provide free services in drug management. Concurrently, the medical insurance scheme was further expanded with the National Essential Drugs List and medical insurance drug reimbursement catalog now including tuberculosis drugs. Multidrug-resistant (MDR) tuberculosis diagnosis and treatment coverage was added to the New Rural Cooperative Medical Scheme and critical illness coverage was added to the Health for Poverty Alleviation program with the objective of increasing patient care.

始终坚持科技创新与合作，不断注入新活力。

Committed to scientific and technological innovation, interagency cooperation, and best practices.

国家层面设立重大科技专项，全面提升结核病防治科研能力。一批批具有自主知识产权的诊断技术陆续投入使用，治疗方案不断优化。创新患者管理模式，结合家庭签约服务，应用互联网工具，提高患者服药依从性。重视国际交流与合作，不断学习借鉴国际先进技术，同时推广中国特色的成功经验。

Major specialized R&D programs were established at the national level to comprehensively improve tuberculosis research capabilities. Numerous new diagnostic techniques with proprietary IP and improved treatment regimens were deployed, innovative patient management models were reinvented, and home-based care services were utilized. Internet tools were used to improve patients' treatment adherence. Advanced technologies and best practices were adopted through international exchanges and cooperation while China's experience with Chinese characteristics were shared.

立足现在、展望未来，中国始终坚持以人民为中心的发展思想，坚持预防为主的卫生与健康工作方针，将健康融入所有政策，履行联合国可持续发展目标承诺，加快推进终止结核病目标的顺利实现！

Looking ahead, China remains committed to human-centered development and a health strategy anchored in prevention. It strives to integrate health into all policies, fulfill the UN Sustainable Development Goals, and accelerate progress towards ending tuberculosis.

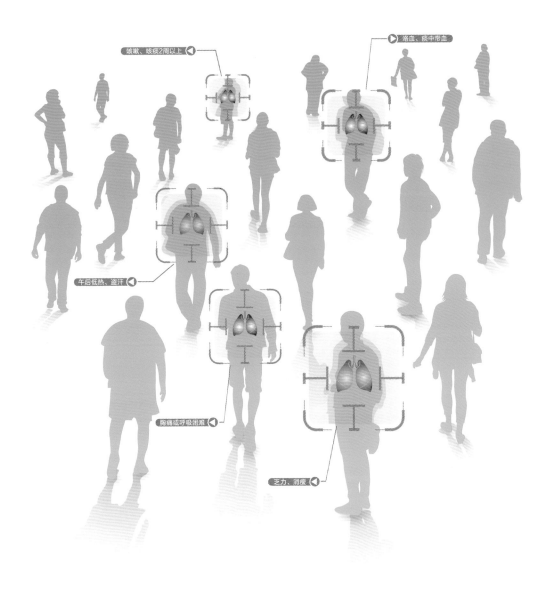

用法律法规强化结核病管理
STRENGTHENING TB MANAGEMENT
WITH LAWS AND REGULATIONS

2004年，国务院修订了《中华人民共和国传染病防治法》（以下简称《传染病防治法》），将肺结核作为乙类传染病管理，确定了疫情报告、通报和公布制度，保障了患者健康权益，为结核病防治工作提供了坚实的法律保障。2013年，卫生部修订了《结核病防治管理办法》，强化了以患者为中心的工作原则，明确了各机构在结核病防治工作中的职责，细化了工作流程，规范了防、治、管各环节的具体措施。

In 2004, the State Council amended the *Law of the People's Republic of China on the Prevention and Control of Infectious Diseases* (hereinafter referred to as the *Law on the Prevention and Control of Infectious Diseases*) which managed pulmonary tuberculosis as a Category B infectious disease. The amendment established an epidemic reporting, notification and disclosure system in addition to codifying patients' health rights and providing a solid legal foundation for tuberculosis prevention and control. In 2013, the Ministry of Health revised the *Administrative Measures for the Prevention and Control of Tuberculosis,* which further clarified the patient-centered principle, defined the responsibilities of different institutions in TB prevention and control, streamlined the workflow and standardized the protocols for prevention, treatment and management.

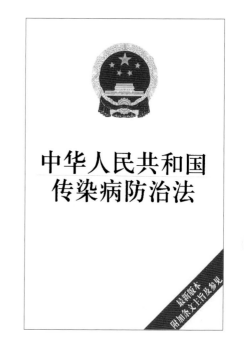

中华人民共和国
传染病防治法

最新版本
附加条文主行政参见

缩短报告时限减少结核传播

Shortened the reporting time to minimize transmission risk

修订后的《传染病防治法》进一步完善了疫情报告和公布制度，要求医疗机构发现疑似肺结核或者确诊肺结核患者应当在24小时内进行网络直报，缩短了报告时限、增加了疫情透明度，对早发现、早诊断、早治疗肺结核，控制结核病传播，具有十分重要的意义。

The amended *Law on the Prevention and Control of Infectious Diseases* further improved the epidemic reporting and disclosure system and required health institutions to report suspected or diagnosed TB cases within 24 hours through an online system. Increased transparency and a shortened diagnosis-reporting timeframe were instrumental in improving the detection, diagnosis and treatment of TB and mitigating the TB transmission risk.

健全防治体系提供全程管理服务

Improved the prevention and control system and enabled full-cycle management

为了更好地对结核病患者提供全面医疗服务，结核病诊断治疗工作由疾控机构转向了定点医疗机构。《结核病防治管理办法》对承担结核病防治工作的相关机构职责进行了界定，形成了疾控机构承担疫情监测及规划管理、定点医疗机构承担诊断治疗、基层医疗卫生服务机构承担居家服药管理的全方位为结核病患者服务的防治体系，保证了防治工作规范、有序开展。

To enable comprehensive health services for tuberculosis patients, TB diagnosis and treatment responsibilities shifted from CDCs to designated medical institutions. The *Administrative Measures for the Prevention and Control of Tuberculosis* defined the responsibilities of relevant institutions responsible for tuberculosis prevention and control. The measures was also put in place a prevention and control system with full-cycle TB patient services including epidemic surveillance and programmatic planning by the CDCs, diagnosis and treatment by designated medical institutions, and home-based drug management by primary healthcare providers. This ensured the standardization and orderly implementation of TB prevention and control plans.

优化预防措施保护人民健康权益

Improved preventive care and ensured patients' rights and interests

肺结核防治相关法律法规详细规定了承担肺结核防治工作的相关机构在肺结核的预防、患者发现、登记、报告中的要求和工作程序，以及肺结核的诊断治疗等工作中的责任，也明确了肺结核患者的权利和义务，既保障了肺结核患者得到有效的治疗和关爱，减少歧视，也保护了健康人群远离结核病威胁，充分显示了以人为本的理念，保护了人民群众的健康权益。

The TB prevention and control laws and regulations specify the requirements and protocols for prevention, case detection, patient registration, and reporting, as well as diagnosis and treatment responsibilities of the relevant stakeholders. They also define the rights and obligations of TB patients, ensuring that they receive effective treatment and care without discrimination. Furthermore, the laws and regulations protect healthy people from the threat of tuberculosis infection. This fully demonstrates a human-centered approach for protecting people's rights to health.

用规划绘制结核病防治蓝图

DEVELOPING A BLUEPRINT FOR TB CONTROL WITH THE NATIONAL PLANNING

为加快推进健康中国建设，进一步减少结核病危害，国务院办公厅先后印发了三个全国结核病防治规划。三个规划立足不同时期，顺应结核病防控特点和医疗卫生体制改革新形势，为中国结核病防治绘制了一张宏伟蓝图。三个规划明确了"政府负责、部门合作、社会参与"的工作原则，强化政府组织领导，在中国结核病防治不同阶段发挥着重要的纲领性作用。

To accelerate progress towards the Healthy China vision and further minimize the public health impact of tuberculosis, the State Council General Office issued three national tuberculosis prevention and control plans. Targeting different periods and recognizing the evolution of tuberculosis control priorities and health system reform, the three plans presented an ambitious blueprint for tuberculosis control in China. The three plans clearly defined the working principles of "government accountability, inter-agency cooperation, and social engagement", which strengthened government leadership and served as important guidelines for different phases of tuberculosis prevention and control efforts in China.

《全国结核病防治规划（2001—2010年）》

提出加强省、地、县三级结核病防治网络建设，实现以控制传染源为中心的现代结核病控制策略（DOTS）全覆盖的目标。

The National Tuberculosis Prevention and Control Plan (2001-2010) proposed a strengthening of the three-tiered (provincial, prefecture and county level) network construction for tuberculosis prevention and control with the goal to better control the infectious disease at the source through achieving full coverage under the DOTS strategy.

《全国结核病防治规划（2011—2015年）》

提出逐步构建疾病预防控制机构、定点医疗机构和基层医疗卫生机构"三位一体"的防治服务体系，实现减少结核病发病和死亡的目标。

The National Tuberculosis Prevention and Control Plan (2011-2015) proposed to gradually build the "3-in-1" TB prevention and control system consisting of CDCs, designated medical institutions and primary healthcare organizations to achieve the goal of reducing TB incidence and mortality.

《"十三五"全国结核病防治规划》

针对终结结核病目标，提出了发病率下降到58/10万的具体目标，强化以患者为中心，实现防、治、管无缝衔接。

The National 13th Five-Year Plan for Tuberculosis Prevention and Control proposed the goal of ending tuberculosis and the specific target of reducing the incidence rate to 58/100,000. This goal emphasized patient-centered principle and seamless integration of prevention, treatment and management services.

中国政府针对结核病防治工作发布的专项规划，成为防治工作的纲领性文件

TB prevention and control plans issued by the Chinese government as guiding documents

用经费保障结核病防治稳步推进
FUNDING TB CONTROL FOR STEADY PROGRESS

中央转移支付地方经费设立结核病防治重大公共卫生项目，经费从2001年的4 000万元增加到2019年的16.8亿元，主要用于为患者筛查和一线抗结核病药品提供补助，开展疫情监测和处置、质量控制、能力建设等工作，2001—2019年累计投入123.7亿元。

The central government set up a critical public health program comprised of transfer payments to local governments for tuberculosis prevention and control. The funding source, which grew from RMB 40 million in 2001 to RMB 1680 million in 2019, is mainly used to subsidize patient screening and first-line tuberculosis drugs as well as TB surveillance and response, quality control, and capacity building, among other activities. Between 2001 and 2019, this funding source has provided RMB 12.37 billion to support these efforts.

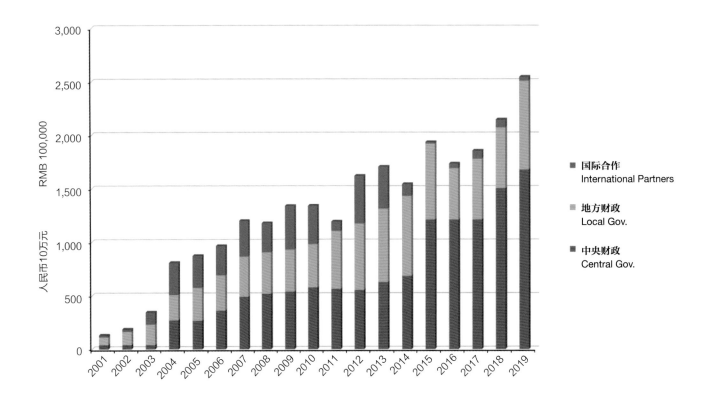

国家基本公共卫生服务项目

Basic public health service program

2015 年，结核病患者管理纳入国家基本公共卫生服务项目，用于患者发现和治疗管理等，每年投入 5.7 亿元，2015—2019 年累计投入 28.5 亿元。

In 2015, the National Basic Public Health Service Program began covering tuberculosis patient management. The program primarily funds patient identification and treatment management, operating with an annual budget of RMB 570 million. Between 2015 and 2019, a cumulative total of RMB 2.85 billion was invested.

地方政府投入

Local government spending

地方政府投入逐年增加，主要用于实验室建设、督导、培训、健康教育等方面，2001—2019 年累计投入 85.9 亿元。

Local government spending increases annually and is generally used to support laboratories, supervisions, training, health education and other activities. Between 2001 and 2019, local governments invested RMB 8.59 billion.

国际合作

International cooperation projects

中国相继引进多个国际合作项目，成为政府投入的有力补充，2001—2019 年累计引入 36.8 亿元。

China has introduced a number of international cooperation projects, which served as a supplement to the inputs of the government. Between 2001 and 2019, a total of RMB 3.68 billion was introduced.

实现结核病疫情持续下降
CONTINUING TO REDUCE TB PREVALENCE

通过各项防治措施的有效实施，中国实现了结核病疫情水平的持续下降，在2010年提前实现了结核病患病率和死亡率双下降50%（在1990年基础上）的联合国千年发展目标结核病控制目标。据估算，2019年中国结核病发病率为58/10万，不到全球平均水平的1/2（130/10万），发病率每年以约3.2%的幅度下降，明显高于全球1.7%的年平均下降幅度。2019年中国结核病死亡率已下降到2.2/10万，远远低于全球16/10万的平均水平。

Thanks to the effective implementation of various prevention and control measures, China has witnessed a continued retreat of the tuberculosis epidemic. In 2010, China achieved the MDGs of halving the prevalence and mortality of tuberculosis (on 1990 basis) ahead of schedule. It is estimated that the incidence of tuberculosis in China in 2019 was 58/100,000, less than 1/2 of the global average (130/100,000). The tuberculosis incidence rate has dropped by approximately 3.2% every year, significantly faster than the 1.7%reduction in the worldwide average. By 2019, China's tuberculosis mortality rate had dropped to 2.2/100,000, far below the global average of 16/100,000.

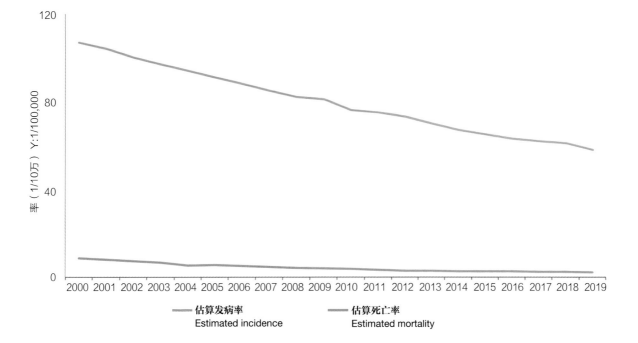

第二章

患者救治
医者仁心

Chapter 2

Promotion of
Early Diagnosis,
Treatment and
Care

中国结核病防治工作
"一切以患者为中心"，
通过患者发现、治疗、管理、关怀等方面
实现全方位为结核病患者服务。

The tenet of tuberculosis prevention and control
in China is to put "patients first in everything we
do", and to provide comprehensive services for
tuberculosis patients through case detection,
treatment, management and care.

多途径发现患者
Detected cases in multiple ways

提高大众对结核病的认知，一旦出现可疑症状，立即就医。对结核病高危人群开展主动筛查，提高发现率。中央财政为结核病可疑症状者进行X线胸片和痰涂片检查提供补助。同时推广使用分子生物学快速检测技术和数字化胸部影像学检查，提高诊断准确性。加强医务人员培训，及时识别结核病可疑症状者，做到及时诊断、及时报告。

Public awareness campaigns were conducted to educate the populace on TB prevention and encouraged them to seek medical advice if they developed symptoms. Active screening for high-risk groups of tuberculosis was conducted to increase detection rate. The central government provides subsidies for X-ray and sputum smear microscopy examination for suspected cases of tuberculosis. At the same time, the use of the molecular biology rapid diagnosis test and chest X-ray digital imaging examinations helped increase diagnostic accuracy. Medical staff were trained to better recognize the symptoms of tuberculosis for timely diagnosis and reporting.

规范化诊疗服务
Standardized diagnosis and treatment services

2001年开始在不同项目地区，为结核病患者免费提供一线抗结核药品，2005年起中央转移地方项目向全国免费提供一线抗结核药品。通过督导服药，提高治疗依从性和治疗效果。2012年卫生部印发《肺结核门诊诊疗规范》、肺结核的临床路径等规范性文件，加强诊疗工作质控，规范诊疗服务，提高诊疗质量。

Starting in 2001, first-line tuberculosis drugs were distributed free of charge to tuberculosis patients in different project areas. Starting in 2005, first-line tuberculosis drugs were provided free of charge throughout the country with funds from the central government's transfer payment program. Supervision of drug administration was implemented to improve treatment adherence. In 2012, the Ministry of Health issued the *Protocols for Outpatient Diagnosis and Treatment of Pulmonary Tuberculosis Patients* and the clinical pathway of tuberculosis, among other prescriptive documents to strengthen quality control of diagnosis and treatment, standardize diagnosis and treatment services, and improve the quality of diagnosis and treatment.

全程管理及关怀

Manage end-to-end patient treatment and care

2015 年，将结核病患者健康管理纳入国家基本公共卫生服务项目，推行家庭医生签约服务制度，把患者关怀融入到健康管理工作中。随着医疗保障制度覆盖面不断扩大，筹资水平逐步提高，其在结核病防治工作中发挥着越来越大的作用，耐多药结核病纳入新农合重大疾病保障，政策范围内报销比例达 70% 以上，部分地区将结核病纳入门诊特殊病种，提高保障水平，切实降低患者医疗负担。针对结核病患者多为贫困人群，一些地区为患者提供了交通、营养补助或营养早餐，同时辅以有效的心理支持和疏导，努力做到不遗漏、全方位关爱患者。

通过一系列举措，2001—2019 年中国发现并成功治疗了 1 440 多万例结核病患者，患者发现率由 2001 年的 35% 提高到目前的 91%，患者治疗成功率自 2001 年以来一直保持在 90% 以上。

In 2015, the National Basic Public Health Service Program added tuberculosis management coverage and a family doctor scheme to integrate patient care into health maintenance. With the further expansion of medical insurance coverage and the gradual increase in funding, the program has played an increasingly important role in the prevention and control of tuberculosis. Multi- drug resistant tuberculosis was included under the critical illness protection section in the New Rural Cooperative Medical Scheme with 70% or above reimbursement levels for qualified claims. In some areas, tuberculosis was included in the special diseases category for outpatient care to increase the level of protection and reduce patient burden. As most TB patients are poor, travel and nutrition allowances (or nutritious breakfast) were provided to patients in some areas, supplemented by effective psychological counseling support to meet the social determinants of health and ensure comprehensive care.

Thanks to the above-mentioned initiatives, some 14.4 million tuberculosis patients were diagnosed and successfully treated in China between 2001 and 2019.The case detection rate has increased from 35% in 2001 to 91% today. The successful treatment rate has remained above 90% since 2001.

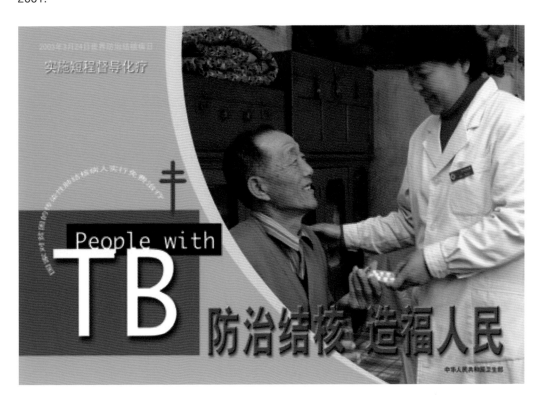

新诊断技术，为我们赢得时间
TIME WON BY THE NEW DIAGNOSTIC TECHNIQUES

让每一位结核病患者早确诊、早治疗，就是为他们赢取战胜病痛、获得重生的宝贵机会。从X线胸片和痰涂片镜检、到痰培养和药物敏感试验、再跨步到今天快速发展的分子生物学检测技术和数字化影像诊断手段，我们一直奔跑在让结核病的诊断时间缩短、再缩短，让诊断结果精准、再精准的路上！

Early diagnosis and early treatment for TB patients provide them with a valuable opportunity to regain health and productivity. From X-ray and sputum smear microscopy to sputum culture and drug susceptibility testing, and now today with rapidly evolving molecular biology detection technology and digital imaging diagnostics, we have been on the road to further shortening the time to diagnose TB and making the diagnosis more accurate.

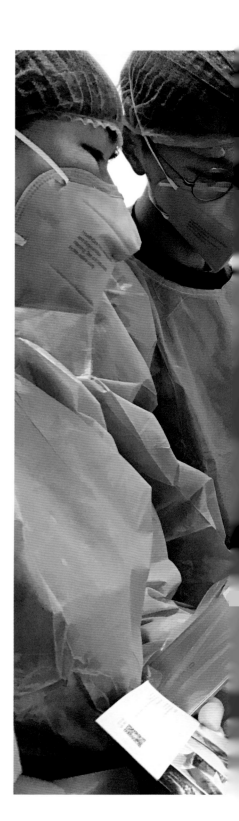

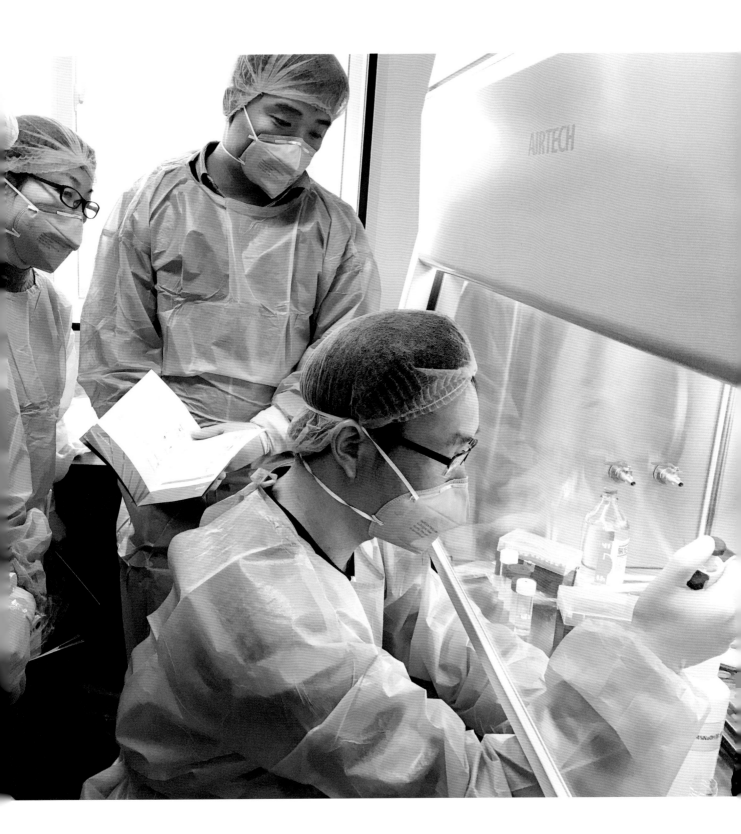

50多岁的农民郑大叔近来总是咳嗽、咳痰、胸闷，到医院检查时医生给他做了X线胸片，结果提示可疑肺结核，需要马上做进一步检查。检验科的李医生用了最新的检测设备为郑大叔做检测，3小时后就拿到了结果，这在以前是根本不可能的。以前要做痰涂片，为了确定最佳治疗方案还需要做痰培养+药敏试验，但这个结果需要等2~3个月的时间。那时，李医生还需要花费很长时间向患者解释"为什么要等这么久？"现在不用解释了，检测结果几个小时就出来了，李医生觉得这设备简直是医院诊断结核病的又一件利器。自从有了它，工作效率大增，关键是确诊结核和药敏检测一次完成，为郑大叔这样的患者赢得了及早治疗的时间，也减少了传染他人的概率。

Uncle ZHENG, a farmer in his 50s, always coughed and expectorated recently. He went to visit the doctor, who then asked him for a chest X-ray. The results suggested he had suspected pulmonary tuberculosis, and the testing for confirmation was needed immediately. Dr. LI of the clinical laboratory used the latest equipment to do the test for Uncle ZHENG and got the results three hours later, which was impossible before. In the past, sputum smear microscopy and drug susceptibility tests had to be done to develop the optimal treatment plan, which took 2-3 months. At that time, Dr. LI had a long time to explain to the patients why it took so long to get the result. Now, without any explanation, the test results came out in a few hours, and Dr. LI thought this equipment was really a great device for diagnosing tuberculosis. Since then, the work has been greatly efficient, esp. tuberculosis confirmation and drug susceptibility test can be done at once, which allows for early treatment of patients like Uncle ZHENG and reduce their risks of further infection.

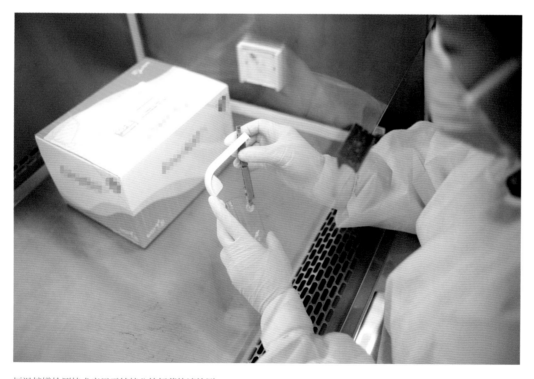

恒温扩增检测技术应用于结核分枝杆菌快速检测
Thermostatic amplification for rapid detection of mycobacterium TB

基因芯片检测技术应用于耐多药结核病快速检测
Gene chip detection for rapid identification of MDR-TB

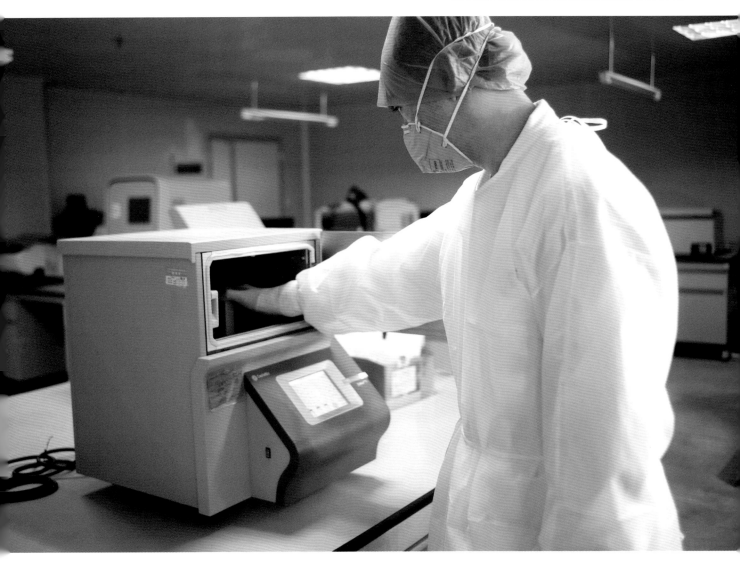

目前，全国各地正在大力推广结核病分子生物学诊断新技术，在设备投入、实验室建设和人员培训等方面下大力气，按照"十三五"规划要求，东中部地区和西部地区将分别有80%和70%的县（市、区）具备开展结核病分子生物学诊断的能力，将有更多患者从新技术中获益。

New molecular diagnostic tests are currently being promoted across the country, accompanied by strong investments in equipment, labs, and personnel training. In accordance with the 13th Five-Year Plan, 80% and 70% of the counties (cities and districts) in the eastern, central regions and western regions will be equipped to run molecular diagnosis tests for tuberculosis, bringing benefits to more patients.

只有坚持，才能治愈

DRUG ADHERENCE TO CURE TB

结核分枝杆菌顽固无情，治疗之路漫长艰辛，中断治疗后果严重，转成耐药菌将更雪上加霜。专业的随访指导、温暖的关怀支持是患者战胜疾病的原动力。6~8个月的服药治疗，是用坚持和信心赢得身体的康复，也赢得了自己新一段的美丽人生！

Mycobacterium tuberculosis is stubborn and ruthless. The road to a cure is long and arduous. The consequences of treatment interruptions are severe, which may resulted in drug resistance and make the treatment even more difficult. Professional follow up and attentive support keeps the patients motivated towards overcoming the disease. Continuous drug administration for 6-8 months requires persistence and confidence to win the recovery and a new period of beautiful life!

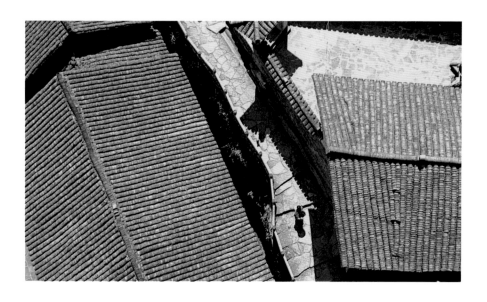

今天，张凤萍（化名）在县结核病定点医院进行最后一次复查，痰菌连续阴性且肺部空洞已闭合，医生说已达到肺结核临床治愈标准。

ZHANG Fengping (pseudonym) had a final tuberculosis treatment follow-up examination at the county TB designated hospital. Her sputum microscopy results were consistently negative and her lung cavity closed. The doctor said she was clinically cured of pulmonary tuberculosis.

走在古镇的街道上，她的心情格外好，这里是有着300多年历史的湘西土家族苗族自治州，这里随处可见秀美风光和古老建筑，这里是中国精准扶贫的首倡之地，也是凤萍的家乡。她没有直接回家，而是要到乡镇卫生院看刘医生，一起分享这个好消息，是在刘医生的鼓励下她才完成了规范治疗。

Fengping felt so great, walking in the streets of the ancient town, in the Tujia and Miao Autonomous Prefecture of West Hunan, with a histroy of more than 300 years. This is her hometown, with beautiful scenery and ancient buildings everywhere, and also the same place where China began the program of targeted poverty alleviation. Fengping decided to see Dr. LIU in the township clinic and share her good news before heading home. Thanks to Dr. LIU's encouragement, Fengping completed the standardized TB treatment.

一年前凤萍被确诊为肺结核，当时的她吓得慌了神。面对凤萍糟糕的情绪，刘医生耐心安慰她："得了肺结核并不可怕，但一定要坚持把药吃好！"随后刘医生帮她联系定点医院，还帮她理清了所有的减免政策。

When Fengping was diagnosed with pulmonary tuberculosis a year ago, she was scared. Dr. LIU patiently calmed her down by saying, "Having pulmonary tuberculosis is not the end of the world, but you must not stop taking the medicine before you get well!" Then Dr. LIU helped contact the designated TB hospital and had her application for treatment subsidies sorted out.

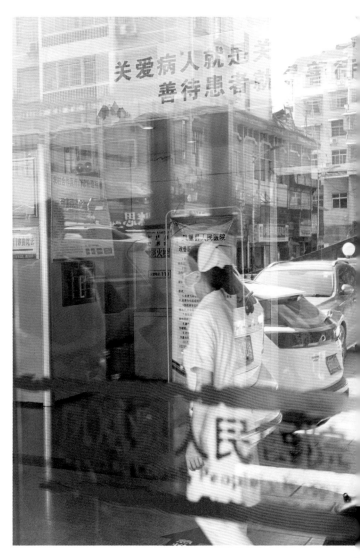

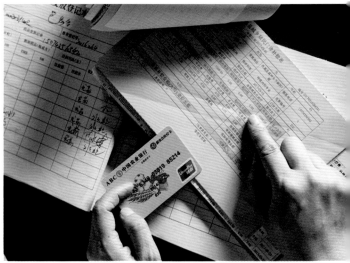

很快凤萍开始了6个月的居家治疗。其间刘医生定期上门随访，每次都是"送药到手、看服到口，记录再走"。凤萍说，起初有些不好意思，吃个药还让人看着，后来慢慢明白了，督导服药是治好病的关键。

Fengping soon started a six-month home-based treatment during which Dr. LIU visited her regularly, each time "delivering the medicine to her hand, seeing her to take the medicine orally, and logging it before leaving". At first, Fenping was embarrassed being watched taking her pills. Over time through, she realized the medication supervised was key to cure the disease.

吃了两周抗结核药后，凤萍的咳嗽症状果然好多了，随着工作的忙碌她渐渐把吃药的事忘了，觉得少吃一两次药也没什么大碍。没想到，刘医生来家里做访视的时候发现了这个情况，严肃地批评了她："你要是不好好吃药，病治不好，还容易产生耐药，要是耐药了，就不是现在这个治法了，一治就得将近两年，还不一定治得好，你愿意吗？难道想让全家老小跟着你受连累么？"

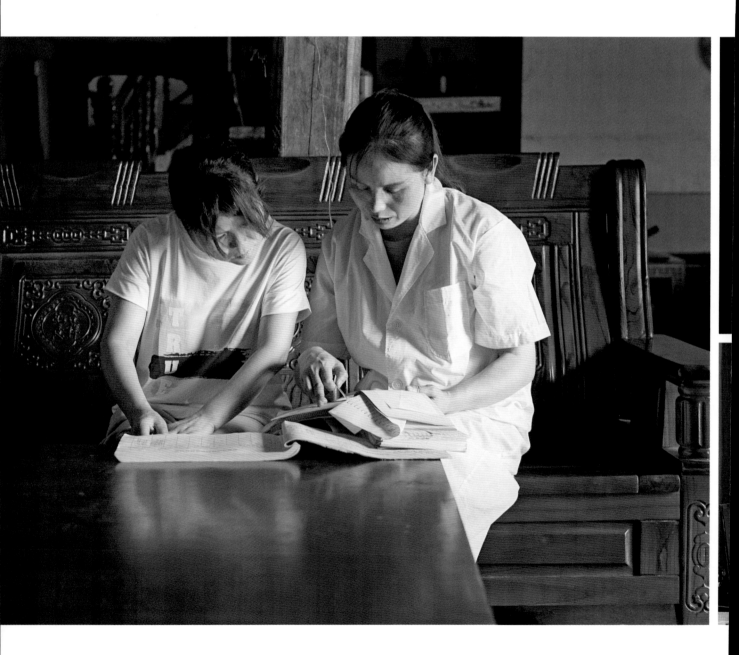

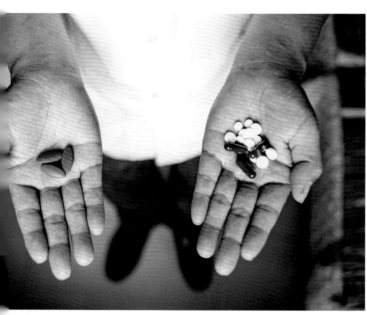

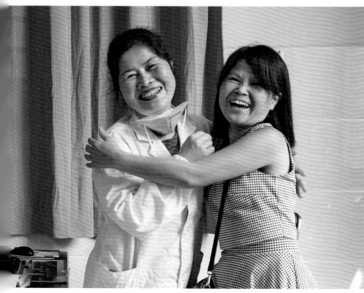

After taking the TB drugs for two weeks, Fengping's cough was greatly reduced. But as she became busy with her work, she sometime forgot about her medicine, and thought that it didn't matter if she didn't take them once or twice. Dr. LIU found the problem in the follow-up visits and warned Fengping seriously, "If you keep skipping your medicine, you won't get well. You may even develop drug resistant tuberculosis. If that happens, the treatment wouldn't be this simple. It would take nearly two years, or even get worse and you may never be cured. Would you take the risk like that? Do you want the whole family to get the same trouble as you have?

风萍记住了医生的话，从那以后她一次也没落过服药。半年后，风萍的肺结核治愈了！风萍喜极而泣，感激地拥抱了医生，她又可以打工养家了。

Fengping remembered what Dr. LIU said. Since then, she didn't miss her medicine, even once. Six months later, Fengping's pulmonary tuberculosis was cured! She shed tears of joy and hugged Dr. LIU gratefully. She is able to work again to support her family.

为了改善患者服药依从性，抗结核病药品已经从最初的散装药、板式组合药品，改进为固定剂量复合制剂（FDC），患者以前每天需要服用一大把药品，现在只需要服用几颗即可。

In order to improve patient treatment compliance, tuberculosis drugs have been changed from bulk drugs and blister pack drugs to fixed-dose combination (FDC) formulations. Patients no longer have to take a large cocktail of drugs, but rather just a few pills a day.

患者关怀，每个环节都要想到做到

CARE AND SUPPORT IN EVERY STEP OF THE THERAPY

贫困人群是受结核病影响的重要群体，有的家庭因结核病而导致贫困。各地政府高度关注民生，多渠道筹资解决结核病患者的诊疗和医疗救助等问题，并将这些举措固化成政策。社会组织也凝聚大爱与善心，为结核病患者提供救助和心理支持。多方力量汇聚成为关爱和帮扶贫困结核病患者的坚强堡垒！

The poor are more susceptible to tuberculosis and tuberculosis can further impoverish a family. With people's livelihoods in mind, local governments are mobilizing funds through multiple channels to solve problems such as TB diagnosis and treatment and medical relief. Such practices are also being codified into policies. Social organizations too are rallying resources to provide relief and psychological support for TB patients. Together these stakeholders are building a strong fortress of care and support for poor TB patients.

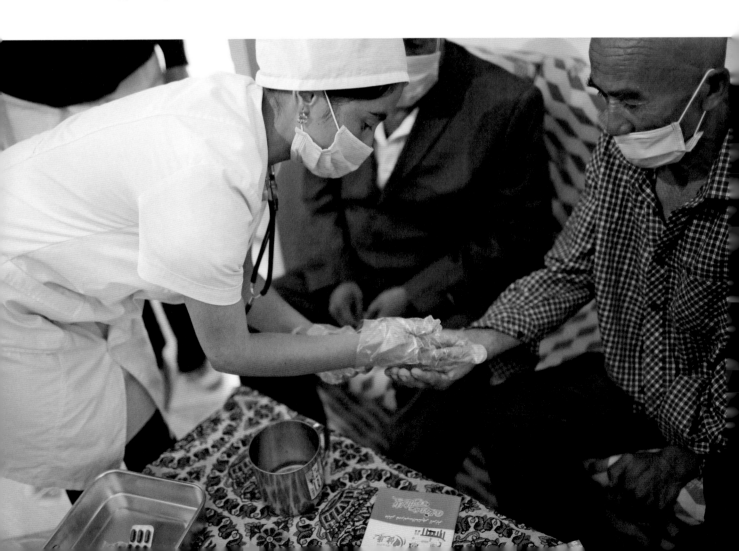

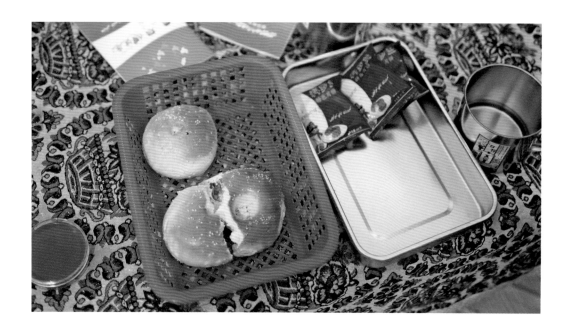

别小瞧了喀什这顿免费早餐
Benefits of free breakfast in Kashgar

在新疆喀什地区疏勒县洋大曼乡且克勒村卫生室里，村医阿依努尔·奥布力喀斯木正在准备集中服药点患者的早餐，包括牛奶、鸡蛋还有馕。他说加强营养，规律服药才能保证治疗效果，而结核病患者多是穷人，营养状况不佳，这一顿免费早餐，可以帮助患者更好地恢复，但要享用这顿早餐，必须配合服药，这些药也都是免费的。

In a village clinic in Shule county, Kashgar prefecture in Xinjiang, the village doctor – Aynur Aubulikashmu– is preparing breakfast for patients visiting the central drug administration station. Each pack includes milk, egg, and nan bread. He says that improving nutrition and taking the drugs regularly can make the treatment effective. Most TB patients are poor and undernourished. This free breakfast can help patients recover better, but to enjoy the breakfast, the patients must first take the drugs which are also free.

67岁的图尔苏·艾买提（化名）是且克勒村来领取营养早餐的患者之一，他家距离村卫生室仅有几百米，走路不到5分钟。他说自己非常愿意去服药点，不仅可以按时服药还可以增加早餐营养，和村医以及病友们说说话，了解结核病的防治知识、最新政策，还能够缓解心理压力。

A 67-year-old, Tulsun Amat is one of the patients coming to collect his nutritious breakfast. He lives less than 5 minutes away, only a few hundred meters, from the village clinic by foot. He says he likes visiting the drug administration station, since not only can he take the pills on time, but he can also have the nutritious breakfast, talk to the village doctor and other patients, gain knowledge of TB prevention and control, be advised of the latest policies, and alleviated of some psychological stress.

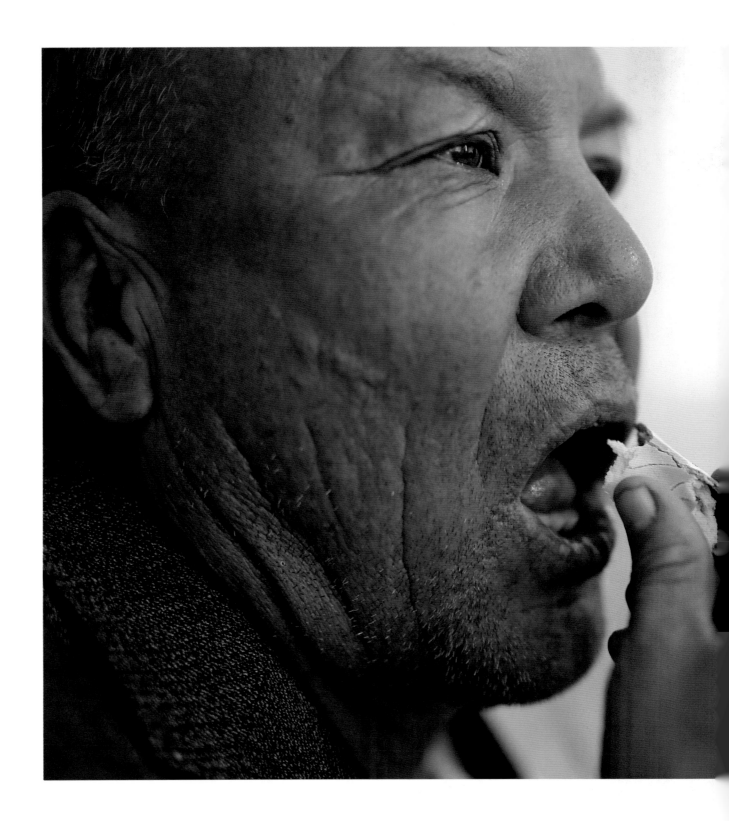

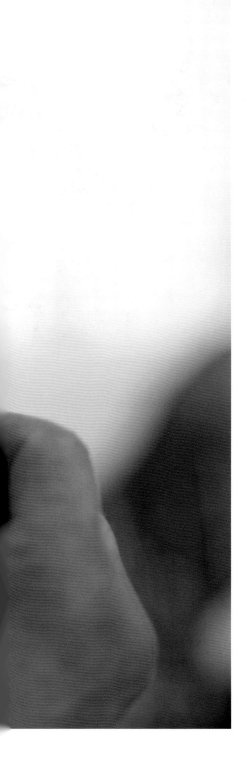

2017年喀什在全地区各县（市）对不具有传染性的患者在村级服药点全面推行"集中服药+营养早餐"的治疗模式。可不要小瞧了喀什的这顿免费早餐。每次早餐前，服药患者需要签字、按手印登记，确保记录真实有效，溯源可查。采用这种督促患者服药的方法虽然简单，却十分奏效，也深得患者的支持。从2014年试点实施，到2017年在全区推广，喀什地区各县共设置了2 300多个集中服药点，目前已经累计有60 000余名患者享受了免费的营养早餐。

In 2017, Kashgar prefecture rolled out the treatment model of "centralized drug administration + nutritious breakfast distribution at the village level" for non-contagious patients in all counties (cities). This is not merely a free breakfast, patients need to sign and fingerprint to ensure that the record is authentic, reliable, and traceable before the breakfast. Simple as it is, urging patients to take their medicine this way works very well and has been warmly received by the patients. From the pilot implementation in 2014 to the promotion in 2017, more than 2,300 centralized drug administration stations have been set up in counties across Kashgar, and more than 60,000 patients have access to free nutritious breakfasts.

正可谓：患者关怀，想到更要做到！

When it comes to patient care, we must think creatively, and more importantly, we must deliver!

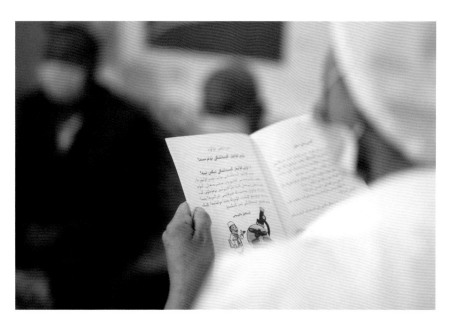

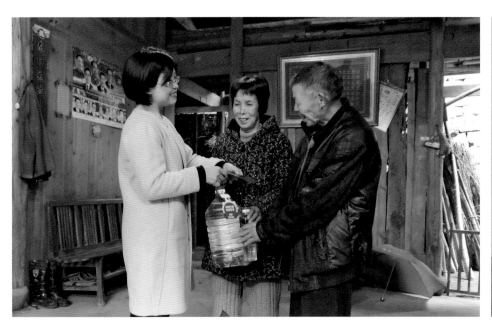

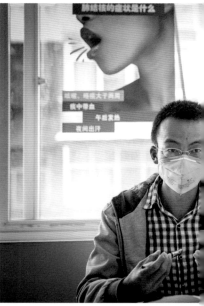

政策保障 降低患者诊疗费用
Costs of diagnosis and treatment reduced by policy support

近年来，为减轻结核病患者的诊疗负担、避免结核病患者出现家庭灾难性支出，国家和各地政府出台了一系列减免政策，降低患者负担，解决患者的后顾之忧。河南省、湖北省当阳市、浙江省桐乡市等地实施肺结核门诊单病种付费政策，提高了门诊报销比例，降低了诊疗费用；上海市，吉林省，浙江省，宁夏回族自治区，江苏省镇江、连云港，安徽省池州等地实施了"医保先行，财政兜底"的做法，则是对肺结核患者提供从诊断到治疗全程的医疗保障，让患者自付比例减少到最低。

In recent years, in order to reduce the burden of tuberculosis diagnosis and treatment of patients, and avoid disastrous family expenditures, the state and provincial governments have introduced a series of relief policies. Henan province, Dangyang (Hubei province), and Tongxiang (Zhejiang province), and other places, have adopted the case-based payment model for pulmonary tuberculosis outpatient services, increased the reimbursement rate for outpatient care, and reduced medical bills. Shanghai, Jilin province, ZheJinang province, Ningxia Hui autonomous region, Zhenjiang and Lianyungang (Jiangsu province), and Chizhou (Anhui province) have introduced the practice of "medical insurance first, and fiscal subsidy for those without insurance" to ensure TB patients can receive the necessary care from diagnosis to treatment and minimize their out-of-pocket expenses.

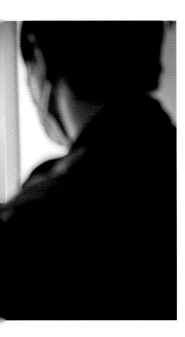

社会关爱 给贫困患者送去温暖
Social support provided to the poor TB patients

为减轻农村贫困结核病患者的经济负担，各地将患者关怀与健康扶贫、精准扶贫相结合，动员社会力量参与，为结核病患者提供更细致、更暖心、更贴心的生活救助和经济支持。

To alleviate the financial burden by poor TB patients in rural areas, patient care has been aligned with local efforts of health for poverty alleviation and targeted poverty alleviation. Social resources have been mobilized to provide more detailed, thoughtful and heart-warming living assistance, and financial support to TB patients.

心理支持 助患者一臂之力
Importance of psychological counseling

小程（化名）是"57天地"的志愿者，同时也是结核病治愈患者，共同的体会和经历让他和患者的心更接近，今天他要跟刚确诊肺结核的阿军（化名）进行一对一的咨询，他说其实结核病患者最怕的有两件事，一是治不好，二是花钱多。所以，他每次都会拿自己成功战胜结核病的例子开导这些新病友，告诉他们只要坚持按时服药，结核病一定能治好，国家和地方已经出台了不少减免政策，结核病治疗自付比例并不高。

CHENG (pseudonym) is a cured, former tuberculosis patient who volunteers at the 57 Center. Share experiences brings him closer to other patients. Today he would like to have a one-on-one counseling with JUN, who has just been diagnosed with tuberculosis. CHENG says as a matter of fact, TB patients are most scared of two things. The first is that TB may not be curable and the second is that it costs a lot of money. So, each time CHENG assuages their concerns by sharing his personal journey of being cured of tuberculosis and telling them that as long as they stick to the drug regimen, they will surely be cured. Thanks to the many relief programs introduced by the state and local authorities, the out-of-pocket payments for TB treatment is not high.

患者离开时如果露出轻松的表情，小程就会感到无比高兴，这就是他和"57天地"所有志愿者小伙伴们工作的意义。"57天地"的志愿者们秉承"因病相识、真诚互助、科学辅导、共渡难关"的理念，大家互帮互助，交流治病经验、疏导负面情绪，传递有温度的人文关怀和正能量，在战胜结核病的道路上共助一臂之力。"57天地"志愿者关怀组织的经验已经辐射到国内的不少地区。

When patients leave with a smile of relief, CHENG feels extremely happy, which is why he works with all the volunteers at the 57 Center. The volunteers uphold the concept of "knowing each other, supporting each other, providing scientific guidance and overcoming difficulties together", and exchange treatment experience, alleviate negative emotions, and bring more care, and positive energy to help the patients in the fight against TB. The best practices of the volunteers of the 57 Center have now been replicated in other parts of China.

七百多个日夜，斩断耐药结核魔爪

EFFORTS MADE IN FIGHTING DRUG-RESISTANT TB

耐多药结核病是严重的公共卫生问题，其传染性更强，治疗周期更长、往往需要18~24个月，治疗花费更大，需要在诊断治疗技术、患者管理关怀等方面形成更强的合力，才能提高患者康复率、减少耐药菌传播，最大限度地减轻社会危害。

Multi-drug resistant tuberculosis (MDR-TB) is a serious public health problem. It is more contagious, and the treatment cycle is longer, often 18 to 24 months. Treatment costs are higher too. In order to maximize the rate of recovery and minimize the social harm of drug- resistant transmission, MDR-TB requires greater alignment of diagnostic and treatment techniques with patient management and care.

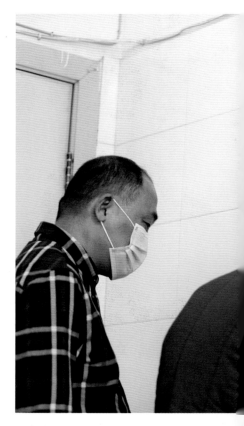

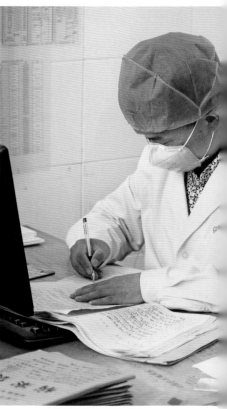

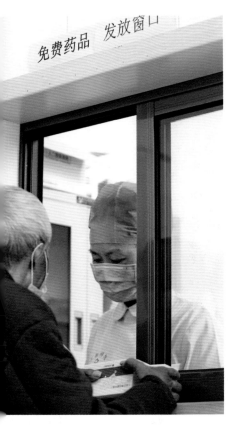

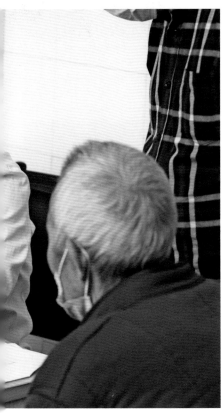

村里的低保户王老汉最近唉声叹气，因为他的肺结核又犯了。这病他以前就得过，药也吃过，但病好一点就不吃了，断了药。这次他把原先的药吃上了，却怎么也不见好，到市定点医院一检查才发现，王老汉得了耐多药肺结核！医生要求他立即住院治疗。

WANG, an old villager living with a low income, has been depressed lately because his pulmonary tuberculosis has relapsed. He had the disease before, and he taken some medicine, but he discontinued treatment when he got better. This time he took the same medicine, but without effect. He visited a TB designated hospital again, and found out that he had MDR-TB! The doctor insisted that he must be hospitalized immediately.

治疗耐多药肺结核，要用二线抗结核药，花的钱更多，治疗时间得两年。王老汉一听，心里打起了退堂鼓，治病的钱从哪来？治还是不治？反正这把老骨头都要交代了。主治医生得知情况后赶紧劝说王老汉，耐多药肺结核一定得治，不治不光自己受累，还可能会传染给家人。耐多药肺结核已经纳入了本省的重大疾病保障，新农合可以报销70%，他是低保户，当地民政部门还可以再报销20%，所以治疗费不用担心。

MDR tuberculosis is treated with second-line drugs that cost more and take two years. WANG wanted to quit the treatment when he heard this, hesitating ".To cure or not?", and thinking "where does the money come from for treatment?" "I might not live much longer". The doctor persuaded Wang, saying that drug-resistant tuberculosis must be treated, not only for his own sake, but also for the sake of his family members. MDR-TB has been included in the major disease insurance in the province. The New Rural Cooperative Medical Insurance Scheme can reimburse 70% and the local civil affairs department can reimburse 20%. So WANG need not worry about the cost of treatment.

听了医生的话，王老汉下定了治疗的决心，七百多个日夜，住院治疗、按时服药、定期复查，一个环节都没有落下，在医生和王老汉的共同努力下，他的耐多药肺结核终于痊愈了！过程虽艰辛，但结果令人欣慰。

Hearing the doctor's words, Wang made up his mind to get treatment. Then, after more than 700 days of hospitalization, scheduled medication, and regular examinations, with the support of the doctor, WANG was finally cured of MDR-TB. The process was strenuous but the results are encouraging.

第三章

体系建设
使命担当

Chapter 3

System Building
of TB Control and
Workforce with
Mission in Mind

中国结核病防治服务体系建设，始终牢记以患者为中心，紧紧围绕控制传染源这一核心措施，紧跟深化医药卫生体制改革步伐，不断强化供给侧改革，努力为患者提供更优质、快捷的防治服务。

Throughout the development of TB control service system, China has followed the patient-centered principle, with the core measure of controlling the source of infection, by deepening reforms of the medical and health care system, further strengthening supply-side reform, and striving to provide better, and more rapid treatment for patients.

多年来，中国结核病防治服务主要以疾病预防控制机构和结核病防治专业机构作为结核病预防、治疗和管理主体，由于当时患者数量较多，而医疗保障覆盖面和水平都较低，该模式既满足了当时患者的基本诊疗需求和药品供应，也有助于全程归口管理和质量控制。2011年以来，随着深化医药卫生体制改革的不断深入，医疗保障覆盖面和水平显著提高，公立医院和基层医疗卫生机构服务能力大幅增强，为满足患者获取更全面的医疗服务需求，结核病防治服务体系逐渐转变为疾病预防控制机构负责疫情监测和规划管理、结核病定点医疗机构负责诊疗、基层医疗卫生机构负责患者随访管理的"三位一体"服务模式。在卫生健康行政部门的统一领导和协调下，各机构职责定位更清晰、服务关怀更全面。

For many years, CDCs and Tuberculosis Dispensaries have undertaken the responsibilities of tuberculosis prevention, control, and management. Due to the large number of patients and the low level of protection provided by medical insurance, this model met the basic medical needs of patients at that time and the supply of drugs and was useful for centralized management and quality control throughout the care cycle. Since 2011, with the deepening of the reform of the medical and health system, the coverage and protection provided by the medical insurance schemes improved significantly, and the capacity of public hospitals and primary healthcare organizations better enhanced, the tuberculosis control service system has gradually shifted to a "3-in-1" model whereby CDCs take ownership for epidemic surveillance and program management, designated medical institutions take charge for diagnosis and treatment, and primary healthcare organizations take responsibility for patient follow-up management, in order to meet the needs of patients to get more comprehensive medical services. Under the leadership and coordination of the health administration, the various actors have further defined their roles and responsibilities, and can deliver more comprehensive services and care.

疾病预防控制机构
CDCs

协助卫生健康行政部门开展结核病防治规划的管理与评估工作；落实患者的追踪、治疗和随访管理；开展结核病信息监测、收集、分析和报告；开展流行病学调查和疫情处置；开展结核病高发和重点人群的防治工作；开展结核病实验室检测和质量控制；开展结核病防治培训，提供防治技术指导；开展结核病防治健康教育工作；开展结核病防治应用性研究等。

Responsibilities: assisting health authorities in management and evaluation of TB control program; patient tracing, managing treatment and follow up; TB information surveillance, case collection, analysis and reporting; epidemiological investigations and epidemic response; prevention and control of high susceptibility and high-risk groups; TB laboratory tests and quality control; personnel training and provision of technical guidance; health education; and applied research on tuberculosis control.

定点医疗机构
Designated medical institutions

负责结核病诊断、治疗及治疗期间的随访检查；负责结核疫情报告和相关信息的登记和上报工作；负责对传染性结核患者的密切接触者进行筛查；负责对患者及其家属进行健康教育等。

Responsibilities: TB diagnosis, treatment, and follow-up during treatment; case reporting; close contact screenings; and health education for patients and their family memebers.

综合医疗机构
General medical institutions

指定内设职能科室和人员负责结核病疫情的报告，负责结核病患者和疑似患者的转诊工作。

Responsibilities:assigning the dedicateddepartments and staff in charge of case reporting, referring patients and suspects to designated medical institutions, and tracking suspected cases.

基层医疗卫生机构
Primary health care providers

负责肺结核患者居家治疗期间的服药管理；负责对辖区内居民开展结核病防治知识宣传；负责对肺结核患者、疑似肺结核患者和有可疑症状的密切接触者进行转诊追踪等。

Responsibilities: supervising drug administration during home-based treatment; disseminating knowledge about TB prevention and control among residents in their areas; referring and tracking confirmed and suspected TB cases in addition to tracing close contacts with TB symptoms.

在积极、稳妥地推进新型结核病防治服务体系构建的同时，中国还在探索、建立结核病分级诊疗和综合管理制度，进一步明确各机构的职责，强化管理，提升服务能力，更好、更全面地为患者服务。

While actively and steadily promoting the development of a new TB prevention and control services system, China is also exploring to establish a grading system for diagnosis and treatment and an integrated management system for TB case management, so as to further clarify the responsibilities of each actor, streamline management, and improve service capacity, to provide better and more comprehensive services to patients.

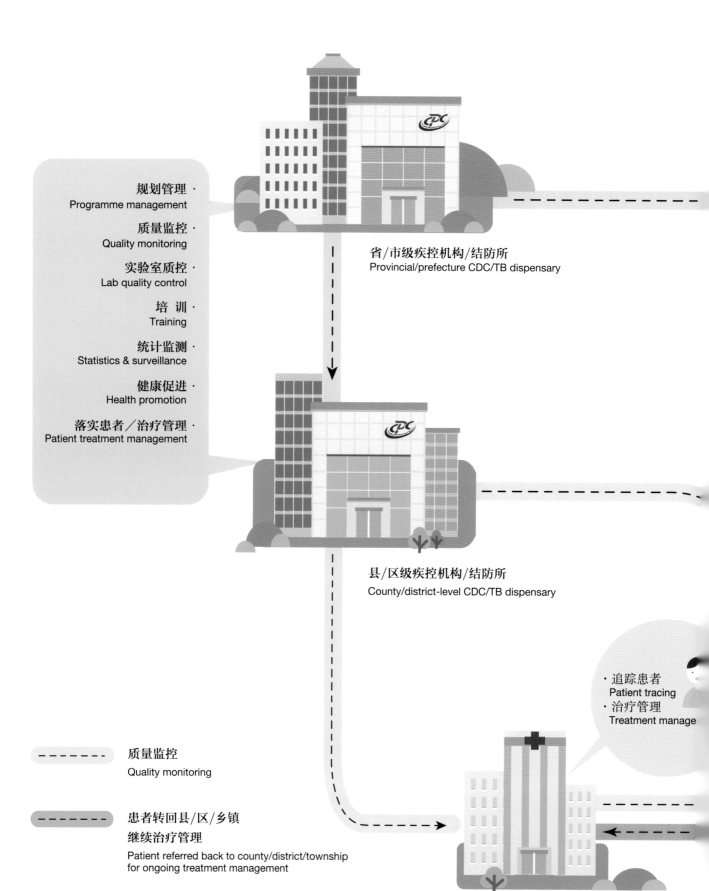

规划管理·
Programme management

质量监控·
Quality monitoring

实验室质控·
Lab quality control

培 训·
Training

统计监测·
Statistics & surveillance

健康促进·
Health promotion

落实患者／治疗管理·
Patient treatment management

省/市级疾控机构/结防所
Provincial/prefecture CDC/TB dispensary

县/区级疾控机构/结防所
County/district-level CDC/TB dispensary

·追踪患者
Patient tracing
·治疗管理
Treatment manage

质量监控
Quality monitoring

患者转回县/区/乡镇
继续治疗管理
Patient referred back to county/district/township
for ongoing treatment management

报告/推荐/转诊
Reporting/Referral/Transfer

乡镇卫生院 ／ 村卫生室
Township hospital/village health clinic

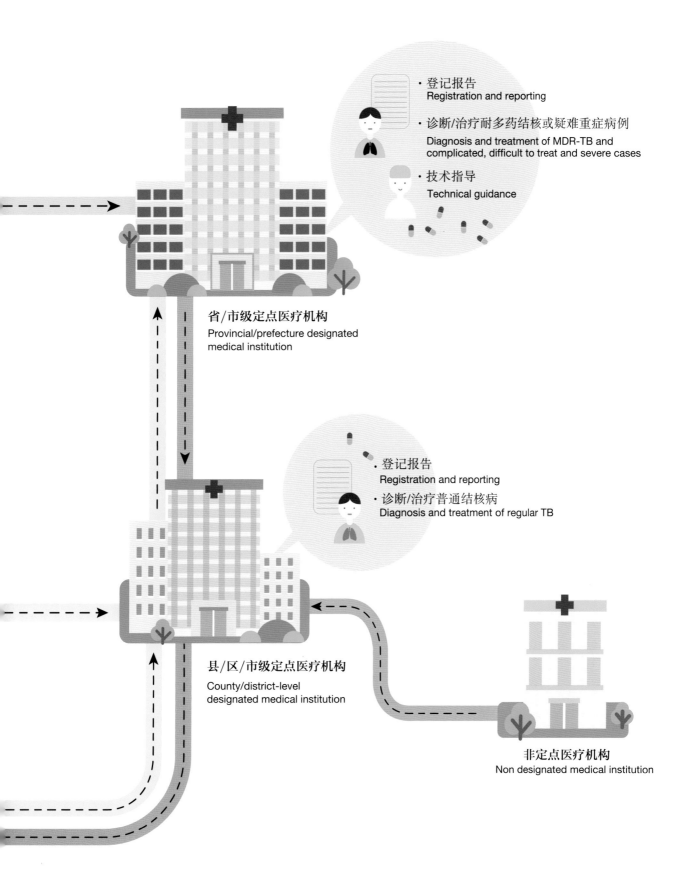

· 登记报告
Registration and reporting

· 诊断/治疗耐多药结核或疑难重症病例
Diagnosis and treatment of MDR-TB and
complicated, difficult to treat and severe cases

· 技术指导
Technical guidance

省/市级定点医疗机构
Provincial/prefecture designated
medical institution

· 登记报告
Registration and reporting

· 诊断/治疗普通结核病
Diagnosis and treatment of regular TB

县/区/市级定点医疗机构
County/district-level
designated medical institution

非定点医疗机构
Non designated medical institution

中国"三位一体"的新型结核病防治服务体系
The"3-in-1"new tuberculosis prevention and control services system

卫生健康行政部门——结防体系的作战指挥部

HEALTH ADMINISTRATION -THE COMMAND CENTER IN THE FIGHT AGAINST TB

加大对建档立卡贫困人口中已治愈、有劳动能力的结核病患者的扶贫开发支持力度，做到精准帮扶、无一遗漏。

Increase targeted support to registered poor populations who are cured of tuberculosis and now have the capacity to work, ensuring no one is left behind.

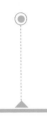

为贫困结核病患者提供人道主义救助，开展健康教育和关爱活动。

Provide humanitarian aid to tuberculosis patients; conduct health education and patient care activities.

指导各地区运用中医药技术方法在结核病诊疗中发挥作用，组织开展中医药防治结核病研究，发挥中医药在防治耐多药肺结核等方面的优势。

Direct each region to use TCM techniques in diagnosis and treatment; organize and conduct research on TCM for tuberculosis control; fully leverage the strengths of TCM in MDR-TB prevention and control.

国务院扶贫办
State Council Leading Group Office of Poverty Alleviation and Development

中国红十字会总会等社会团体
NGOs such as the China Red Cross Society

国家中医药管理局
State Administration of Traditional Chinese Medicine

**国务院
防治重大疾病工作
部际联席会议制度**

国家卫生健康委
National Health Commission

国家发展改革委
National Development and Reform Commission

中央宣传部、国家广播电视总局
Publicity Department of the Central Committee of the Communist Party of China and the National Radio and Television Administration

教育部
Ministry of Education

加强结核病防治基础设施建设，改善防治设施条件。

Strengthen the infrastructure for tuberculosis prevention and control; improve the conditions of the prevention and control facilities.

承担国务院防治重大疾病工作部际联席会议办公室职责，会同有关部门共同组织实施结核病防治规划并开展监督评估；加大贫困地区结核病防治力度，对农村贫困结核病患者进行分类救治；将结核病防治作为传染病防治监督执法的重要内容；协调完善全国结核病防治服务网络和专业队伍；建立健全结核病防治信息管理和共享机制。

Host the office of the State Council Interagency Taskforce on the Prevention and control of Major Diseases; jointly organize and implement tuberculosis control plans and conduct the supervision and evaluation in partnership with other relevant agencies; intensify tuberculosis prevention and control efforts in poor regions; provide circumstance relief to poor rural tuberculosis patients; treat tuberculosis as an important component of supervision and law enforcement for the control of communicable diseases; coordinate and improve the national tuberculosis prevention and control network and professional workforce; establish and improve tuberculosis prevention and control management and information sharing.

开展结核病防治工作公益宣传，普及结核病防治知识。

Conduct public outreach campaigns on tuberculosis prevention and control; raise the awareness about tuberculosis prevention and control.

加强学校结核病宣传教育，落实新生入学体检等防控措施，创建良好学校卫生环境，督导学校做好疫情报告，严防结核病疫情蔓延。

Strengthen tuberculosis education in schools; implement preventive and control measures such as medical examinations at enrollment; create a hygienic environment in schools; supervise school tuberculosis reporting; and strictly contain the spread of tuberculosis.

加强对抗结核药品的审批和质量监管，完善药品质量抽验机制。

Strengthen approvals and quality controls for tuberculosis drugs; improve the process of random quality checks on drugs.

完善医保政策，推行医保支付方式改革，对符合条件的贫困结核病患者按规定给予医保救助，提高结核病患者医疗保障水平。

Improve medical insurance policies; reform payment models under the medical insurance schemes; provide medical insurance assistance to qualified poor TB patients in accordance with regulations; and increase the level of protection for TB patients.

加强口岸结核病防治知识宣传教育，组织各直属出入境检验检疫机构落实口岸结核病疫情监测和管理工作。

Spread knowledge and raise awareness of tuberculosis prevention and control at customs ports; organize directly affiliated entry-exit inspection and quarantine agencies to conduct epidemic surveillance and management of possible tuberculosis outbreaks at ports.

根据结核病防治需要、经济发展水平和财力状况，合理安排补助资金并加强资金监管，保障防治工作开展，切实减轻肺结核患者就医负担。

Sensibly allocate subsidies according to the needs of tuberculosis control, the level of economic development, and availability of financial resources; improve fund oversight to ensure the appropriate conduct of tuberculosis prevention and control expenditures; tangibly reduce the burden on tuberculosis patients.

海关总署
General Administration of Customs

国家市场监督管理总局
State Administration for Market Regulation

国家医疗保障局
National Healthcare Security Administration

财政部
Ministry of Finance

State Council Interagency Taskforce on the Prevention and Control of Major Diseases

科技部
Ministry of Science and Technology

工业和信息化部
Ministry of Industry and Information Technology

公安部、司法部
Ministry of Public Security and Ministry of Justice

民政部
Ministry of Civil Affairs

加强结核病疫苗、诊断试剂、治疗药物和方案等新技术研究，推进科技重大专项等科研项目对结核病防治研究工作的支持；将结核病防治知识宣传纳入科普宣传工作计划。

Strengthen research on new technologies such as tuberculosis vaccines, diagnostic reagents, treatment drugs, and therapies; promote scientific research projects such as major R&D to support tuberculosis prevention and control; feature tuberculosis prevention and control knowledge in science popularization programs.

会同国家卫生健康委对被监管人员开展结核病检查和治疗管理；将结核病防治知识纳入监管场所干警和医务人员的岗位培训和教育内容，纳入被监管人员的入监（所）和日常教育内容。

Work with the National Health Commission to regulate tuberculosis examinations and treatment for the regulated groups; incorporate tuberculosis prevention and control knowledge into job training and education for police officers; and enhance tuberculosis prevention and control knowledge into onboarding and routine trainings for medical personnel at regulated establishments for regulated groups.

组织协调抗结核药品、试剂的生产供应，完善相关产业政策，支持企业加快技术改造，增强抗结核药品创新和生产能力。

Organize and coordinate the production and supply of anti-tuberculosis drugs and reagents; improve relevant industrial policy; support enterprises to accelerate technological upgrades; stimulate innovation and increase production capacity for tuberculosis drugs.

拟定社会救助政策，对符合条件的贫困结核病患者按规定给予基本生活救助。

Formulate social relief policies to provide minimum living allowances for qualified poor tuberculosis patients.

疾病预防控制机构——结防体系的作战参谋部

CDCS - THE JOINT STAFF OF THE SYSTEM IN THE FIGHT AGAINST TB

疾病预防控制机构是公共卫生战线的核心阵营，在结核病防治工作中侦察和作战两不误，疫情关口一马当先，调查处置责无旁贷，但更多的寻常岁月，疾控人员是默默无闻地打拼在基层一线的健康守望者，为百姓带来长久的安宁和健康。

Centers for Disease Prevention and Control (CDCs) are the core for a strong defense of public health. The fight against tuberculosis requires that CDCs have greater efforts to monitor the epidemic, and a swift response to the public health emergency at the frontline and take the immediate action for case investigation. CDCs, work as health guardians to ensure the health and wellbeing of the people.

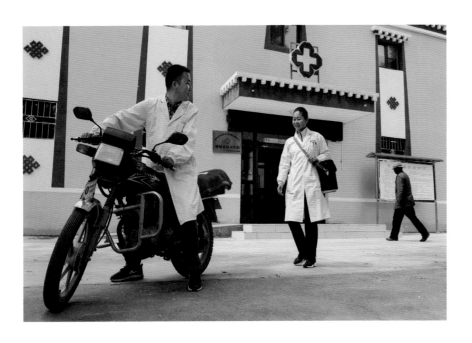

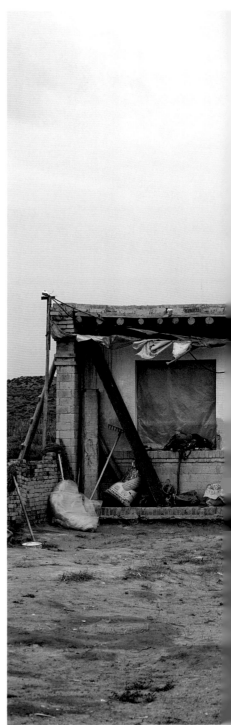

来自青海藏族自治州的拉热措在县疾控中心已工作19年了，这里曾是结核病的
高发地区。十几年来，为保护藏区同胞的健康，拉热措的奔波足迹遍布县里的
大街小巷。

Rajecho has worked at the county CDC in Qinghai Tibetan Autonomous Prefecture
for 19 years. This area used to have a high incidence of tuberculosis, but for
more than 10 years Rajecho has been working up and down the county streets to
protect the health of residents in the Tibetan communities.

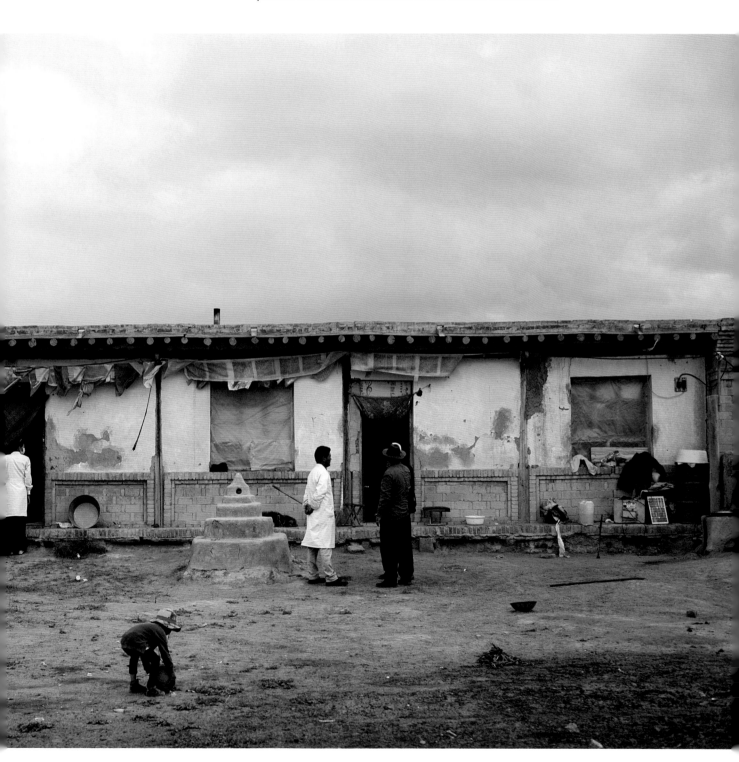

每天一上班，她都要仔细关注结核病信息管理系统的动态变化，做好辖区结核病患者的追踪、随访和管理；出现疑似疫情时，拉热措第一时间会同有关专家赶赴现场进行调查和处置；她还和县医院医生约好经常去开展患者管理、健康教育和感染控制等的技术指导。

Every day at work, she first checks the TB information management system for updates. She traces, follows up, and manages tuberculosis patients in her catchment area. If a suspected TB case is reported, she will rush to the scene with tuberculosis experts for investigation and response. She also works together with the doctors of the county TB designated hospital to regularly provide technical guidance on patient management, health education, and infection containment.

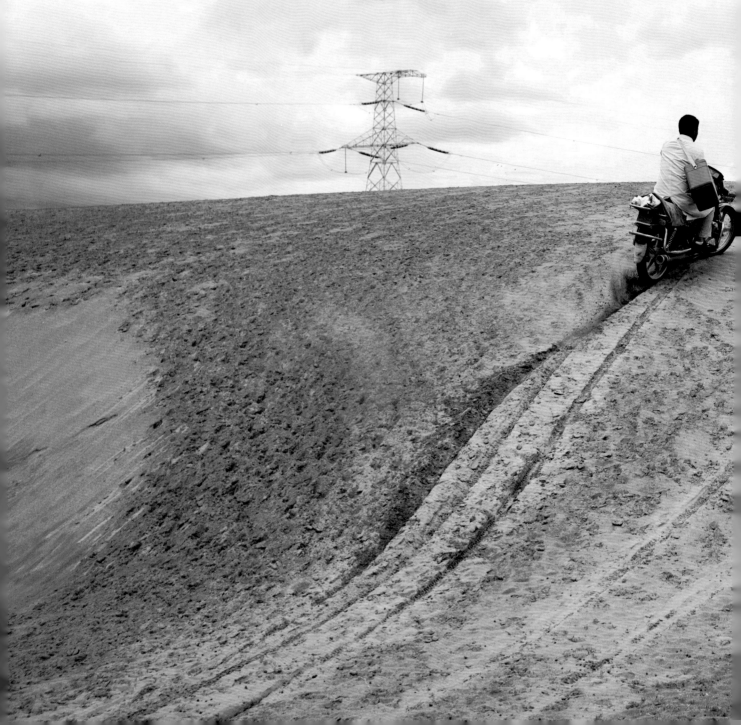

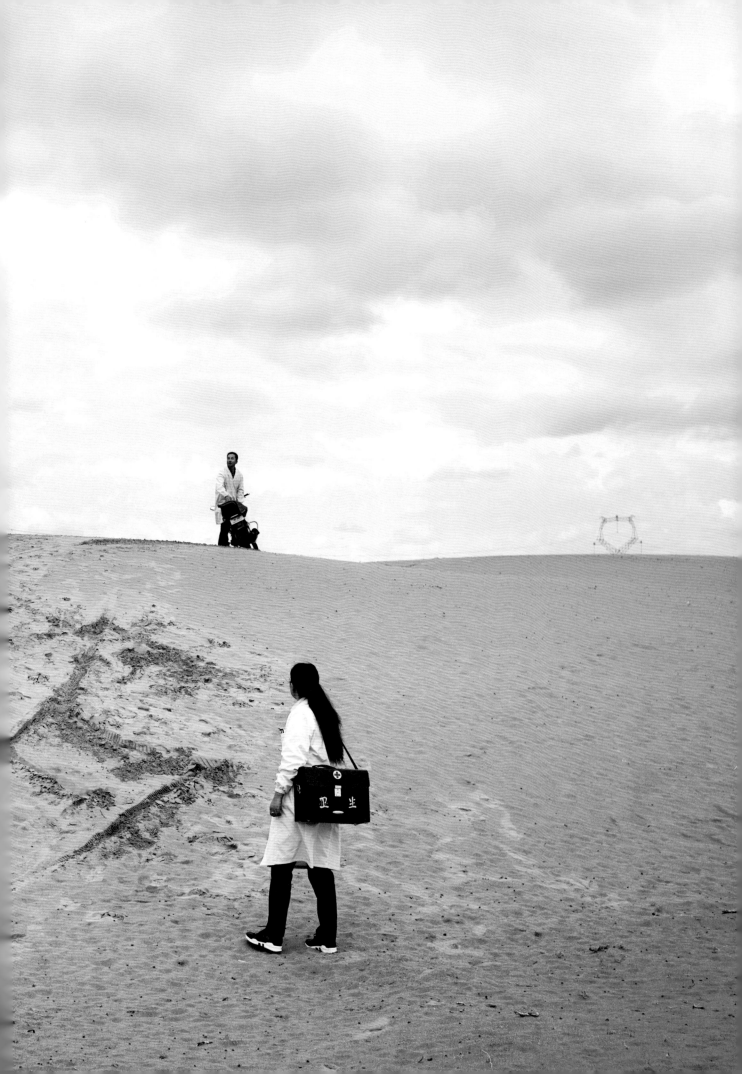

拉热措深知基层疾控机构也要当好卫生行政部门的决策助手，她定期开展结核病信息监测和分析，并把重要结果和工作建议及时地报告给卫生行政部门做参考。

Rajecho is aware that the grassroots CDCs should be a good assistant of the health administration. She regularly monitors and analyses TB information, and reports important findings and recommendations to the health administration department in a timely manner.

这一天，她到乡卫生院与结核门诊的医生汇合，俩人骑上摩托车经过一段沙漠路途再与当地村医集合，他们要一起到牧民家做访视。

That day, she went to meet a doctor from the TB outpatient department of the township hospital, and the two rode a motorcycle through the desert to meet with the local village doctor for follow-up visits to the herdsmen's home together.

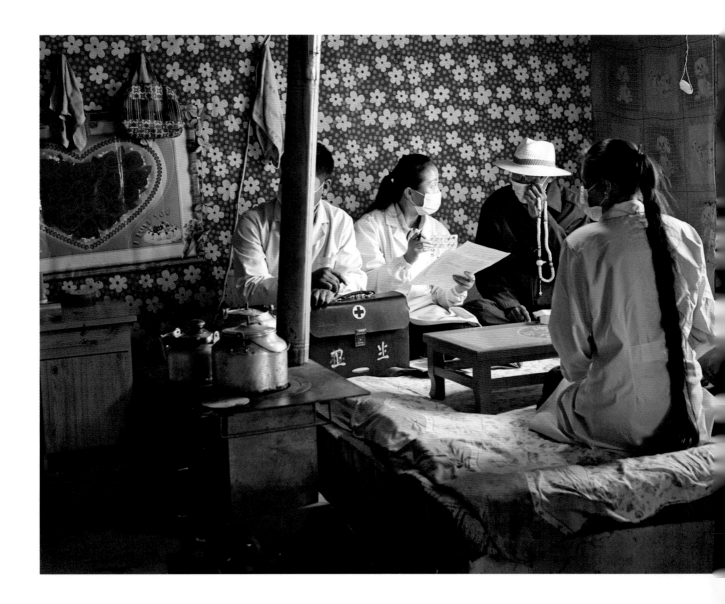

这位牧民1个多月前确诊为肺结核并开始用药，目前处在强化期，按规定拉热措要前去完成督导。在牧民家中，拉热措认真询问并记录他的服药情况，仔细检查了药物剩余与保存情况，分发宣传手册给患者，提醒牧民要注意讲卫生，有问题第一时间找村医。

The herdsman was diagnosed with TB more than a month ago and began to use drugs and currently in an intensive phase of treatment. Rajecho was required to follow up the case. At the herdman's home, Rajecho carefully asked questions and recorded his treatment adherence. She carefully checked the remaining pills and reservation, left the pamphlets to the patient, reminded him of personal hygiene, and advised him to reach out to the village doctor whenever he has a question or concern.

在中国，像拉热措这样的基层疾控工作者很多，他们奔波在结核病防控的主战场，是结防体系作战参谋部的核心兵力，为公众的健康和患者的康复保驾护航。

There are many grassroots CDC workers like Rajecho in China. They are busy and rushing forward at the grassroots level and backbones in the network of TB prevention and control for protection of the people's health, and promotion of patient recovery

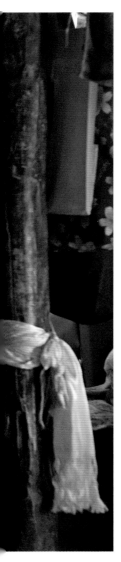
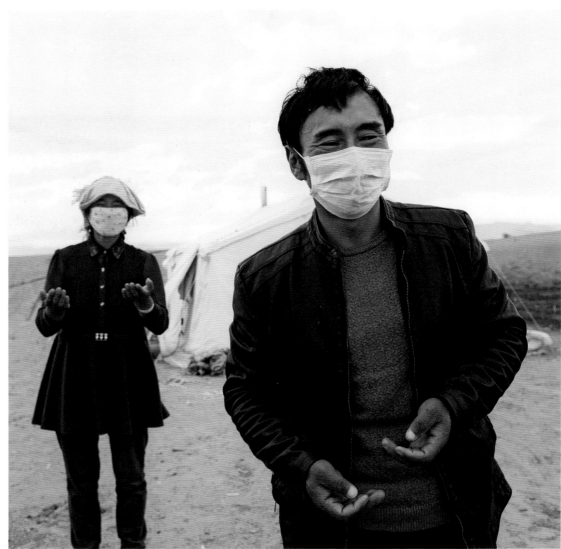

定点医院——结防体系的前沿阵地

DESIGNATED HOSPITALS - THE FRONTLINE AGAINST TB

新型防治服务体系赋予结核病定点医院更神圣的职责，结核病的定点医院除了履行其基本的诊断治疗职责外，还同时担当了结核病预防控制的公共卫生责任。定点医院和疾病预防控制机构在患者发现、诊断、治疗和管理的各个环节拧成一股绳，全力为结核病患者提供更优质的服务。

Tuberculosis designated hospitals play a great role in the new service system. In addition to basic responsibilities of diagnosis and treatment, they also undertake the tasks of public health for TB prevention and control. The designated hospitals work closely with CDCs to provide better services for TB patients in all stages – case detection, diagnosis, treatment, and patient management.

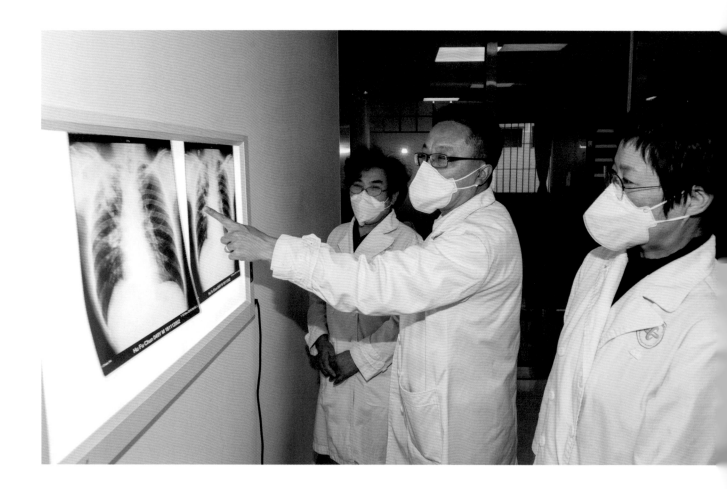

廖医生是县级定点医院结核科的医生。一大早他就接待了一位综合医院转诊过来的肺结核可疑症状者，他仔细查看了医疗本上的记录：咳嗽、咳痰超过两周，伴胸闷、乏力、午后盗汗，X线胸片检查提示可疑肺结核。

Dr. LIAO is a doctor at the TB department of a county designated hospital. Early in the morning. He received a patient referred from a general hospital with suspected TB symptoms. He carefully checked the patient's medical record: cough with phlegm for more than two weeks, chest tightness, fatigue, afternoon sweating, weakness, and chest x-ray examination, indicating suspicious TB.

廖医生对患者进行了详细的问诊，然后让他去做分子生物学检测。廖医生所在的结核门诊有独立院落，与院内其他门诊病区分道通行，避免了患者之间的交叉感染。

Dr. LIAO examined the patient in detail and then sent him for a molecular diagnostic test. Dr. LIAO's tuberculosis outpatient clinic is separate from other parts of the hospital, which is accessible by separate roads to avoid cross-infection among patients.

检测结果提示为普通肺结核。廖医生耐心向患者交代服药要求，这些话他已经重复了不知多少遍，但他知道规律服药对治疗效果至关重要，所以一点也马虎不得。开完处方后廖医生又为患者出具了三联转诊单，告诉他交给社区医院的医生，后续将由他们督导患者完成居家治疗。末了，他还叮嘱患者一定要按时过来复查。

The test result of the patient indicated common pulmonary tuberculosis. Dr. LIAO then patiently advised the patient how to take the medicine. He repeated these words many times as he knew drug adherence is important for the effect of the treatment and the patient must not ignore this. After writing the prescription, Dr. LIAO issued a triplicate referral form for the patient, telling him to deliver it to the doctors at the community clinic, who would then take over the home-based treatment supervision. Finally, he reminded the patient of the follow-up examination on time.

送走了患者，廖医生打开电脑的结核病网络报告系统，将患者的信息填报。鼠标一点，这个患者的信息就会发送到整个网络系统中，疾控中心和社区的医生便可以及时掌握追踪，大家协同一道把患者的治疗管理工作做得严丝合缝。

After the patient left, Dr. LIAO reviewed the TB reporting system on his computer and filled in the patient's information. With one click, the patient's information would be reported via the network, and doctors in the CDC and the local community can keep track of the patient in a timely manner and work together to manage the case.

目前，中国每个县都设有结核病定点医疗机构、每个地市和省级设有耐多药定点医疗机构，充分满足患者诊疗需求。

Currently, every county in China has a designated medical institution for tuberculosis, and every prefecture, city, and province has designated MDR-TB medical institutions to fully meet patients' needs for diagnosis and treatment.

结核病定点医疗机构职能
Functions of designated medical institution for tuberculosis control

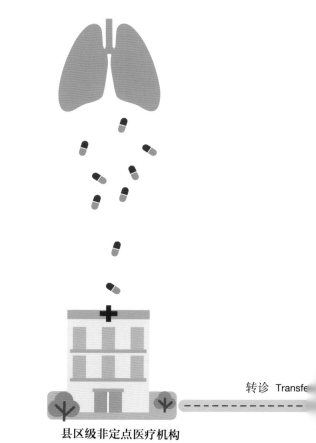

转诊 Transfe

县区级非定点医疗机构
County/district-level non-designated medical institution

就诊 Consultation

就诊 Consultation

就诊 Consultation

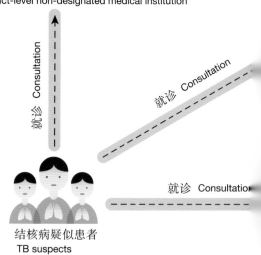

结核病疑似患者
TB suspects

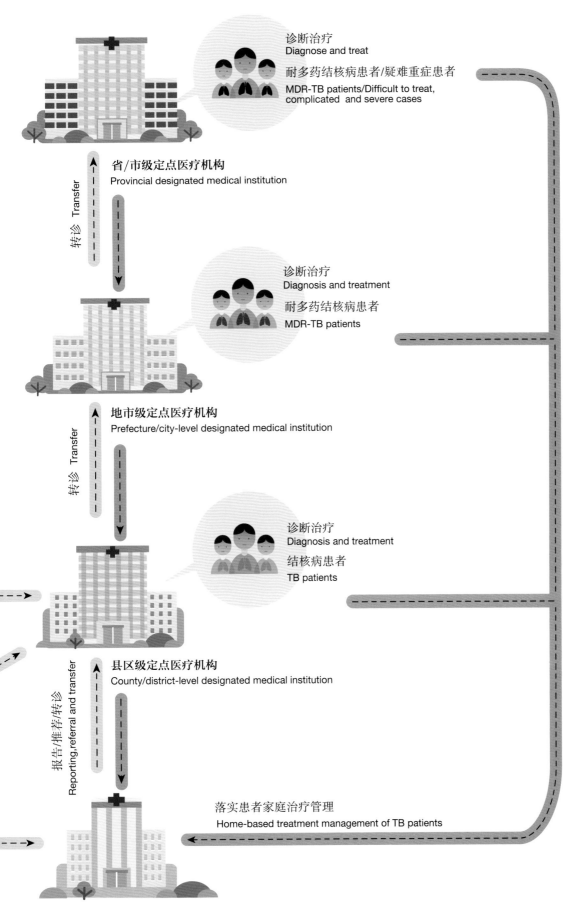

诊断治疗
Diagnose and treat

耐多药结核病患者/疑难重症患者
MDR-TB patients/Difficult to treat,
complicated and severe cases

转诊　Transfer

省/市级定点医疗机构
Provincial designated medical institution

诊断治疗
Diagnosis and treatment

耐多药结核病患者
MDR-TB patients

转诊　Transfer

地市级定点医疗机构
Prefecture/city-level designated medical institution

诊断治疗
Diagnosis and treatment

结核病患者
TB patients

报告/推荐/转诊
Reporting,referral and transfer

县区级定点医疗机构
County/district-level designated medical institution

落实患者家庭治疗管理
Home-based treatment management of TB patients

基层医疗卫生机构
Primary health care provider

基层医疗卫生机构——结防体系的防护网

PRIMARY HEALTH CARE PROVIDERS–THE PROTECTIVE NETWORK AGAINST TB

基层医疗卫生机构是为结核病患者提供治疗管理，同时侦察和推荐结核病可疑者及早检查、明确诊断的最接地气的公共卫生网络机构。基层社区和乡间村落的医疗卫生工作者年复一年、日复一日、披星戴月地穿行、服务于当地千家万户的老百姓，用专业和便捷构筑起一道人民健康的牢固防线。

Primary health care providers make up a locally connected public health network that provides treatment management for TB patients and identification and referral of suspected cases for immediate examination and clear diagnosis. Year after year and day after day, grassroots health workers in communities and rural villages work diligently to help tens of thousands of local households, and build a solid defense against the disease through their professionalism and accessibility.

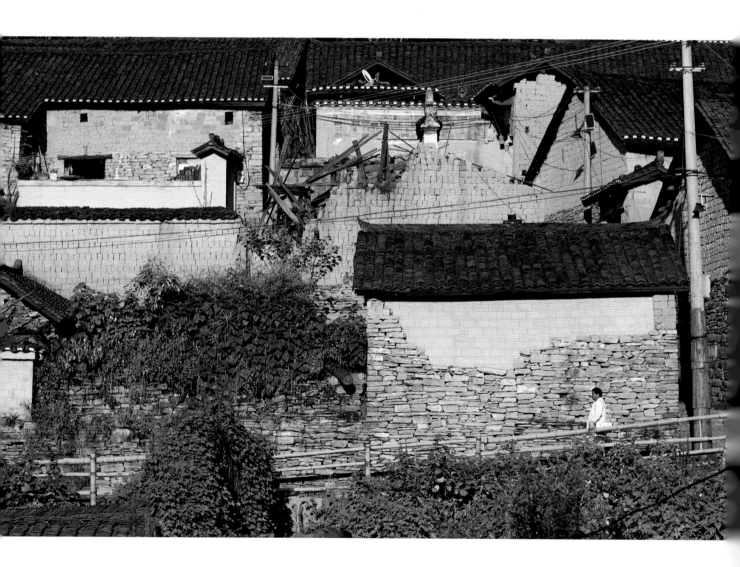

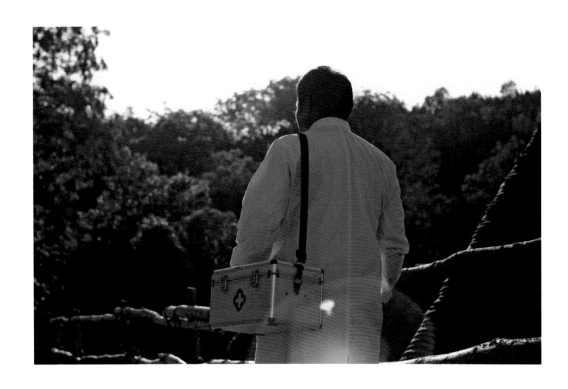

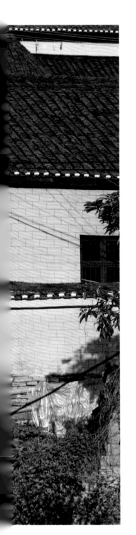

村医——小小螺丝钉，发挥大作用
Village doctors–small bolts that play large roles

中国中部地区某县扭仁村53岁的村医麻孔位做村医38年来，他日出而作，日落而息，精心地照料着村民们的健康。他的工作主要是结核病患者日常治疗管理，除了结核病，他还要负责全村400多人的慢病管理。麻孔位今天要到村东头去督导老陈服药，这已经是老陈服药的第53天了。老陈总是颇有感触地说：要不是麻医生跟着，他真是坚持不下来天天吃这些药片。

In Niuren, a small village in a central province of China, MA Kongwei, a 53-year-old village doctor, working for 38 years, takes good care of the villages' health cautiously and conscientiously. His main responsibility is the daily treatment management of TB patients. In addition, he is also responsible for chronic disease management for more than 400 people in the village. MA is going to the eastern part of the village today to supervise an old patient named Chen for his medication. This is already the 53rd day of CHEN's treatment. CHEN always emotionally says, had it not been Dr. MA's supervision, he really couldn't have kept taking the pills every day..

麻孔位说看着患者好好吃药是自己的责任，他还有一个心愿就是等村里再也没有结核病了，他就把健康教育列为自己的工作重点，毕竟预防是基础、是关键！

Dr. MA said that it was his duty to have his patients take their medicine as required. His wish is to see his village free of tuberculosis someday in the future, and at that time, he will focus on health education, as he knows that prevention should be the first!

中国有许多像麻孔位一样的一线工作人员，落实解决了结核病防治工作最后一公里的问题。

China has many health workers like Dr. MA, who help so solve the "last mile problem" of tuberculosis control.

社区医院，家门口的服药点
Community clinics, accessible and convenient for drug administration

每天早晨，患有肺结核的阿强（化名）都会步行10分钟到离家最近的社区医院去服药，他已经坚持4个月了。

Every day in the morning, QIANG, a pulmonary tuberculosis patient walks 10 minutes to the nearest community clinic to take his TB medicine. He has been on the treatment for 4 months.

为了方便结核患者服药，深圳（广东）按照患者服药控制在步行15分钟内到达的要求，在全市设立了600多家督导服药点。每位患者均在医生面视下进行督导服药，做到"看服到口，咽下才走"。

In order to facilitate TB treatment, Shenzhen (Guangdong) has set up more than 600 sites for the patients to take medicine in the city, as it is required that the clinics should be within 15-minute walk. Each patient takes the medicine under the watch of a doctor.

阿强服药所用的一卡通是深圳市肺结核患者的服药ID卡，这张卡可以在任何一家社区督导服药点使用，如果外出办事来不及回家服药，可以在手机APP上查询就近服药点，非常方便。而且电子网络督导管理系统还可以及时掌握辖区管理患者的数量变化、服药情况和不良反应等情况，对患者进行实时动态分析、评估和服务。

QIANG keeps a ID card for his medication in Shenzhen, which can be used in any one of the community sites. If a patient is away from home, he or she can conveniently check the nearest site on the mobile phone app. Additionally, the networked digital supervision and management system can keep abreast of the changes in the number of patients, medication, and adverse reactions, providing real-time dynamic analyses, evaluations, and services to patients.

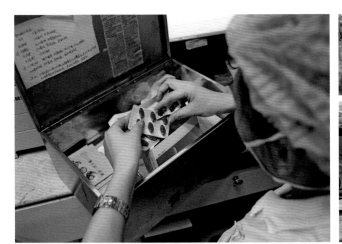
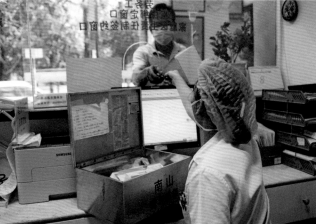
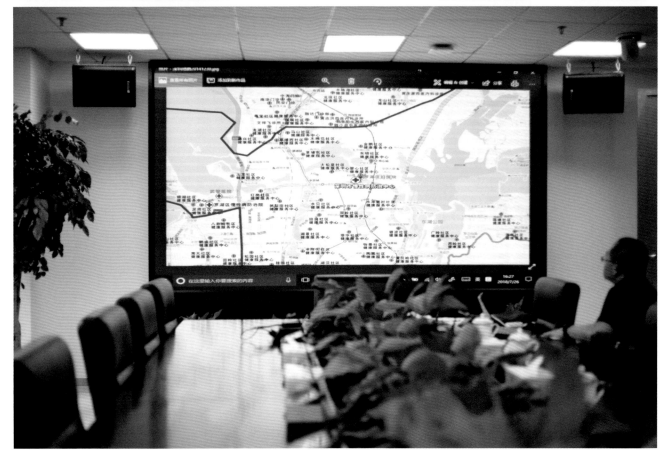

第四章

重点人群
精准施策

Chapter 4

Measures Targeted
to Key Groups
with the Right
Strategies

结核病患者的密切接触者、艾滋病病毒感染者、流动人口、在校学生、老年
人、糖尿病患者等，都是结核病易感人群，针对不同重点人群，需要采取有针
对性的防控措施。

People in close contact with TB patients, people living with HIV/AIDS, migrant
populations, school students, and the elderly are the most vulnerable to TB and
susceptible to infection because of weak immunity. Targeted prevention and control
measures are necessary for high-risk populations.

结核病患者的密切接触者
Close contacts of TB patients

指与具有传染性的肺结核患者直接接触的人员，包括家庭成员、同事和同学等。
自 2006 年开始，全国范围内开展了密切接触者筛查，尽早发现发病的密切接触者，
并及时治疗。

refers to the people who have direct contact with infectious pulmonary
tuberculosis patients, including family members, co-workers, and classmates.
Since 2006, China has conducted close contact screenings across the country,
to detect TB cases among close contacts as early as possible and provide timely
treatment.

艾滋病病毒感染者
People living with HIV/AIDS

艾滋病病毒感染者免疫力受到破坏，容易感染结核菌，造成致命危害。为做好结
核菌 / 艾滋病病毒双重感染防控工作，中国为所有艾滋病病毒感染者和患者提供
结核病筛查服务，在艾滋病流行重点县（市），为结核病患者提供艾滋病病毒筛
查服务。为结核菌 / 艾滋病病毒双重感染患者及时提供治疗与关怀，提高患者生
命质量。

People living with HIV/AIDS suffer from a loss of immunity and are susceptible to
tuberculosis infection, potentially causing fatal harm. In order to prevent and control
TB/HIV co-infection, China provides tuberculosis screening services to all people living
with HIV/AIDS and HIV screening services for tuberculosis patients in key HIV/ AIDS
epidemic counties (cities). The purpose of the screenings is to provide timely treatment
and care to the patients with tuberculosis and HIV/AIDS co-infection, and ultimately
improve their quality of life.

流动人口
Migrant population

流动人口流动性和聚集性强，管理难度大，是结核病防治的重点和难点之一。目
前中国对流动人口的结核病防控采取属地化管理，同时利用信息管理系统做好流

动人口结核病诊断、报告、转诊追踪、信息登记和治疗随访等工作。

The migrant population is mobile, highly concentrated, and difficult to manage, which is one of the top priorities and greatest challenges of tuberculosis control. China currently adopts localized management of tuberculosis prevention and control for the migrant population. At the same time, the internet-based TB reporting and management system are used in diagnosis, reporting, referral and tracking, log information, and follow-up of treatment of the migrant population.

在校学生
School children

结核病防治是学校卫生工作的重点之一。青少年学生学业压力大，教室和宿舍环境人员密集，是结核病防控的重点人群。原国家卫生计生委和教育部联合印发了《学校结核病防控工作规范》，要求全国各大、中、小学校要严把学校结核病防控的五个关口：入学体检关、症状筛查关、疫情报告关、密切接触者筛查关、休学复学关，做到早发现、早诊断、早治疗，以保障学生健康安全。

TB control is one of the priorities of school health. Adolescent students are usually in the environment of the crowded classrooms and dormitories. They are a key group for TB prevention and control. The former National Health and Family Planning Commission and the Ministry of Education jointly issued the *Guidelines for the Prevention and Control of Tuberculosis in Schools,* which require all universities, secondary, and primary schools across the country to strictly adhere to the five checkpoints for TB prevention and control in school: physical examination at admission, symptom screening, case reporting, close contact screening, and suspension and return to school from the sick leave. The purpose of these five points are to protect the health and safety of students by achieving early detection, early diagnosis, and early treatment.

其他重点人群
Other key groups

将结核病筛查与老年人体检、慢病及糖尿病体检相结合，对羁押场所的在押人员开展入监体检、定期筛查、监测，落实结核病患者治疗管理等相关措施。

TB screening is combined with other physical examinations such as check-ups for the elderly, chronic disease patients, and diabetics/physical examination. Physical examinations, regular screening and monitoring are carried out for detainees in the places of detention and relevant measures such as treatment and management of TB patients are implemeted.

重点人群结核病防控工作从强化宣教、主动筛查、预防性治疗、全程管理和贴心关怀等多个维度入手，全面有序地推进，落实预防为主，最大限度地减少人群发病。

The prevention and control of tuberculosis in key groups is achieved through multiple dimensions such as strengthening education, active screening, preventive treatment, whole-course management, and patient care. Such efforts should be advanced in a comprehensive and orderly manner with prevention as the first strategy to minimize the incidence of people.

用好四大法宝，保障外来务工人员健康
THE FOUR TOOLS USED TO PROTECT THE HEALTH OF MIGRANT WORKERS

改革开放 40 余年，推动中国经济的迅猛腾飞，广大的外来务工人员成为推动所在地经济和建设发展的生力军，他们是劳动价值的创造者，但受居住条件、营养状况、工作强度等因素的影响，他们也是容易受到结核病侵袭的对象，关心和保护他们的身心健康、开展健康宣传教育、为其提供全方位的结核病预防控制服务，防范疾病发生，已成为当地责无旁贷的工作任务。

The last 40 years of reform and opening up have seen the rapid development of China's economy. The vast number of migrant workers has become a vital force behind local economic prosperity. They create value through their labor, but they are still vulnerable to tuberculosis infection due to the inadequate living conditions, nutritional status, and work intensity, among other factors. Health promotion and education are essential to protect their physical and mental health, and it is incumbent upon all working in public health to provide them with a comprehensive services of TB prevention and control to minimize TB spread.

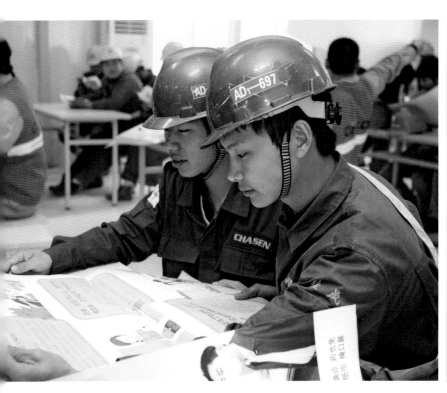
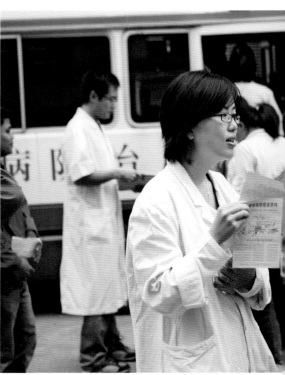

珠江三角洲某市的科技园区，外来务工人员云集，人员结构复杂、流动性大，结核病防控工作难度很高。在当地结核病防治机构的指导和帮助下，用"四大法宝"做到了结核病早发现、早治疗，保障工人健康安全，避免疫情发生。

In a hi-tech park in a city of the Pearl River Delta, migrant workers are gathering – the workforce is a complex mix and the mobility is high. With guidance from the local TB prevention and control agencies, the "four great magic tools" are used to achieve early detection and treatment of tuberculosis, to ensure the health and safety of workers, and to prevent outbreaks.

健康体检是基础
The first is health checkup

新招募的员工先要接受入职体检，在岗的老员工每年要体检一次，合格才能上岗，若发现疑似肺结核患者，会立即安排筛查或转诊。

New employees must first undergo a physical examination upon starting work. Current employees are required to undergo a physical examination once a year. If a suspected pulmonary tuberculosis case is found, screening or referral will be arranged immediately.

带薪病假是后盾
The second is paid sick leave

员工一旦确诊肺结核，持诊断证明，可申请至少3个月的带薪病假，病假期间每月可获1 000多元的生活补助，直到传染性消失后返岗。

Once an employee has been diagnosed with pulmonary tuberculosis, he or she can apply for at least 3 months of paid sick leave by presenting a valid diagnosis certificate. During the sick leave, he or she can receive a living allowance of RMB 1,000+ per month until his or her return to work after he is no infectious.

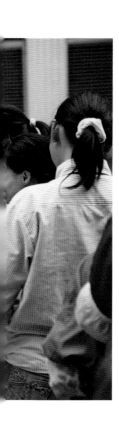

医疗补助是保障
The third is medical benefits

为每位参加职工医疗保险的人员每年门诊报销一定额度医疗费用，可用于支付国家免费项目之外的其他辅助检查、治疗费用。除此之外，持疾病诊断证明也可以向企业申请报销医保报销后的遗留费用。

A certain amount of medical expenses is reimbursed annually by the migrant worker's medical insurance, which can be used to cover the costs of supplementary examinations and treatments in addition to the state's free treatment program. Furthermore, workers can also apply to their employer for reimbursement of the remaining post-medical insurance expenses with a valid diagnosis certificate.

健康宣传是关键
The fourth is health promotion

为提高员工对结核病的认识和自我防护能力，企业会请优秀的健康教育专家深入厂区开展形式多样的健康宣传活动，向广大工人介绍结核病的危害、识别和防护方法。

In order to improve employees' awareness of TB knowledge and their ability to protect themselves, excellent health education experts are invited to carry out various forms of health promotion activities in the factories to introduce the knowledge on the risks of TB and inform workers on how they can protect themselves against TB.

守好五个关口，保障学生健康

THE FIVE CHECKPOINTS SET TO PROTECT THE HEALTH OF STUDENTS

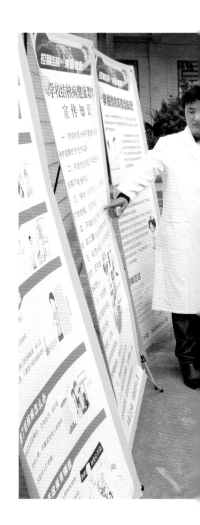

青少年是未来的创造者、民族的脊梁，少年强则祖国强，保护好青少年的健康，就是保护好了民族的未来。学生是容易感染和发生肺结核的群体。校园的居所环境、学生的课业负担、个体的免疫功能、自身的防范意识等因素影响到校园肺结核疫情的发生。不论学校的防病管理、还是学生的个体防护，都需要把好连环关口，保证万无一失。

Young people are the creators of the future and the backbone of the nation. When young people thrive, the motherland thrives too. Protecting young people's health secures the future of the nation. Students as a group are susceptible to TB infection and pulmonary tuberculosis. The campus environment, the student's academic burden, the individual's immune system, and their own awareness of self-protection all have a bearing on the occurrence of tuberculosis at school. No matter of the school's disease prevention management, or the individual protection of students, it is important to maintain the healthcare continuum.

第一关：入学体检关

First checkpoint: medical examination at admission

每年9~10月，某疾控中心结防科的武科长就开启了"5+2"和"白加黑"的工作模式。他要对全市16个乡镇、街道办事处所辖的新生入学结核病筛查工作进行指导。开学第一天，他给学生发了"致学生家长的一封信"，使新生入学结核病筛查工作比往年进行得更加顺利。目前，中国各大、中、小学校及幼儿园，都把结核病筛查纳入入学体检及教职员工体检，若发现疑似患者及时到定点医疗机构进行确诊，同时开展筛查、追踪等后续的管理工作。

Mr. WU, the chief of the TB control division of a local CDC, had his busiest season from September to October each year. He even worked 7 days a week. He was responsible for supervising the TB screening of new students in his jurisdiction of 16 townships, villages, and sub-district offices throughout the city. On the first day of school, he sent out an letter to the students' parents so that the tuberculosis screening with new students could go more smoothly than it had in previous years. All major kindergartens, primary and secondary schools, and universities in China now include tuberculosis screening during the medical examination admission test. Faculty and staff are also tested as part of their medical examination. Suspected cases are referred to designated medical institutions for conformation diagnosis and follow-up management activities, such as screening and tracing, take place simultaneously.

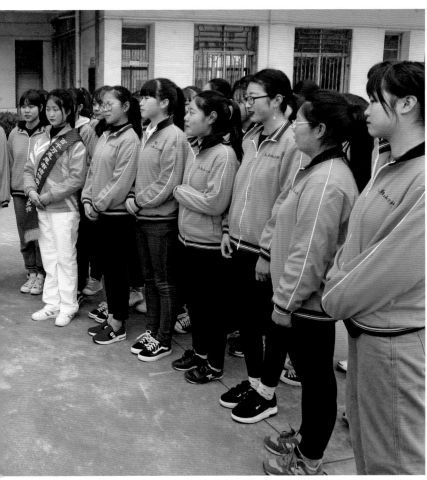
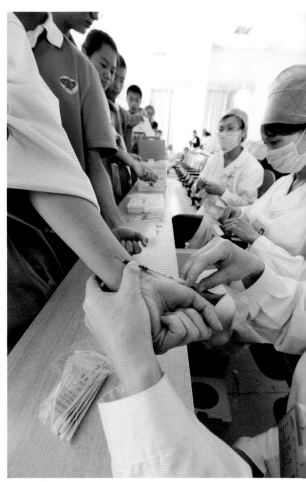

第二关：症状筛查关

Second checkpoint: symptom screening

某小学的校医在得知该校六年级有4名学生同一天因为病假没有来上学，她马上去找班主任老师逐一核定情况：其中1个孩子骨折，1个孩子去看牙医，还有2个孩子有发热、咳嗽的症状。校医立即嘱咐班主任老师跟后2个孩子的家长取得联系，告知他们带孩子尽快去医院检查。下午，班主任老师拿来了这2名学生的检查报告，确认都是普通感冒，悬着的心终于落地了。

When the school doctor at an elementary school found that 4 students in the grade 6 missed school on the same day because of sickness, she immediately went to the head teacher to verify the situation: student A had a bone fracture, student B was at the dentist's office, and students C and D had fever and cough symptoms. The school doctor immediately instructed the head teacher to contact the parents of students C and D and advised them to take their children to the hospital for examination as soon as possible. In the afternoon, the head teacher received the two students' hospital results, which confirmed that they merely had the common cold. The school doctor finally felt relieved.

保障学生健康安全要把好症状筛查关，做好晨检、因病缺勤病因追查及登记、病例报告和疫情监测等工作。

To ensure the health and safety of students, it is important to screen for symptoms, do morning checks, search and register causes of absenteeism, and conduct case reporting and surveillance.

第三关：疫情报告关

Third checkpoint: case reporting

某市重点中学高三3班班主任在一次晨检中发现学生小王（化名）精神萎靡不振，还老咳嗽，她赶紧将情况报告给校医室，校医李医生马上联系了学生家长，建议他到医院检查，最后学生被确诊为肺结核。得知这一情况校医立即拨通了当地疾控中心结核科刘医生的电话，向他报告了情况，他们一直保持着密切的联系。及时的疫情报告为患者的治疗管理和后续的密切接触者筛查打下基础。

During morning check, the head teacher of class 3, grade 3 of of a key high school found that a student named WANG was in low spirits and coughing. She quickly reported it to the school doctor, Dr. LI, who immediately contacted WANG's parents and advised WANG to go to the hospital for an examination. WANG was later diagnosed with tuberculosis. Upon learning about this, Dr. LI immediately called Dr. LIU from the TB control division of the local CDC and reported the case. The doctor had kept in close touch with the student ever since. Timely case reporting provides the basis for patient treatment management and subsequent close contact screening.

第四关：密切接触者筛查关

Fourth checkpoint: close contact screening

疾控中心结核科刘医生得知这所学校学生小王被确诊为肺结核，他片刻不敢耽误，马上联系学校进行密切接触者筛查。

Dr. LIU of the tuberculosis department of the local CDC learned that WANG, a student of the school, had been diagnosed with tuberculosis. Without any delay, he contacted the school to arrange for screening of close contacts.

所有与小王有直接接触的人都需要筛查是否感染肺结核，包括他的家人、同班师生和同宿舍同学。筛查工作有序地进行，结果也很快出来了，发现结核菌素试验强阳性者1人，其余均正常。医生建议强阳性人员接受预防性治疗，从而降低结核病的发病风险。

All those in direct contact with WANG needed to be screened for tuberculosis, including his family members, teachers, classmates, and roommates. Then the screening was carried out, and the results came in quickly. One person was detected with a strong positive tuberculin test while the others were TB negative. The doctor recommended that the person with TB positive must receive preventive treatment to minimize the risk of tuberculosis attack.

从得知情况到完成筛查，只用了两天的时间。面对这个结果，刘医生长长地舒了一口气。把好密切接触者筛查关，才能防止结核病传播，防止疫情出现。

It took only two days for the completion of the diagnosis. Dr. LIU was relieved finally. It is necessary to screen close contacts to prevent the spread of tuberculosis and reduce the risk of an outbreak.

第五关：休学复学关

Fifth checkpoint: suspension and return to school from the sick leave

今天是西藏林芝地区各学校开学的日子，12岁的拉珍（化名）背着新书包高高兴兴地来到学校，要知道她可是一个学期都没有见到同学和老师了，因为她被确诊为肺结核后按照医生的治疗建议办理了休学，休学期间她在家里坚持规范治疗，连续2次痰涂片检查均为阴性，一次痰培养检查也是阴性，所以定点医院给拉珍出具了复学诊断证明，拉珍又可以上学了！

On the first day of school in Linzhi prefecture, Tibet, Lazhen, a 12-year old girl happily arrived at school with her new bag. She had not seen her classmates or teachers for a whole semester because she was suspended from school on doctors' advice after being diagnosed with tuberculosis. During the suspension, she insisted on standardized treatment at home. The sputum smear test was negative for 2 consecutive times, and the sputum culture test was also negative. Therefore, the doctor in the designated hospital gave Lazhen a re-school certificate so that she was happy to go to school again!

把好休学、复学关，是双保障——保障孩子的健康和学习！

Suspension and return to school are a double guarantee for students' health and learning!

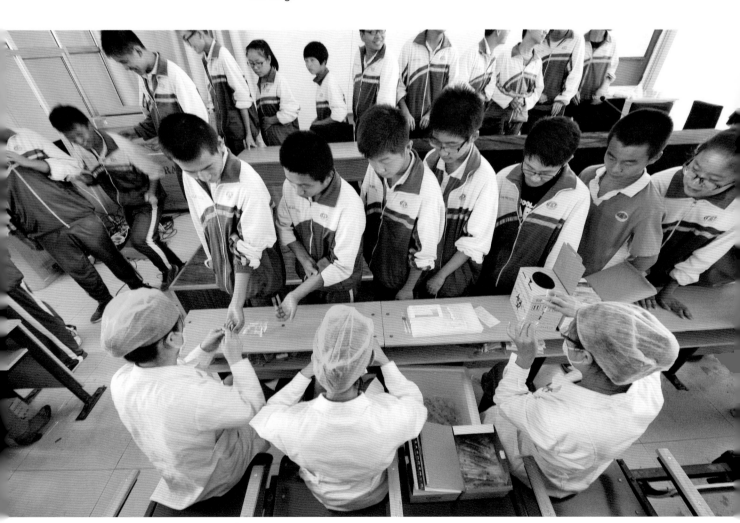

警惕结核病，关爱老年人健康

VIGILANCE AGAINST TB AND CARE FOR THE HEALTH OF THE ELDERLY

老年人因其机体免疫力降低，感染结核菌后易发病，且因症状较隐匿往往就诊不及时，极大地影响到健康水平和生活质量。预防老年人结核病，要主动出击、双管齐下，一方面在健康体检中加入结核病筛查项目，及时发现、立即治疗、尽早治愈；另一方面，利用体检等机会加大对老年人群的结核病防治宣传，不断增强他们的防病意识。

With reduced immunity, the elderly is prone to morbidity after infection with mycobacterium tuberculosis. A further challenge is that symptoms are often less noticeable among the elderly, leading to delayed clinical consultation, which greatly affects their health and quality of life. Prevention requires preactive efforts and two aspects should be paid. The first is to combine TB screening with health checkup to ensure timely detection, immediate treatment, and an early recovery. The second is to use the physical examination and other opportunities to spread knowledge of tuberculosis prevention and treatment among the elderly, to further raise their awareness of disease prevention.

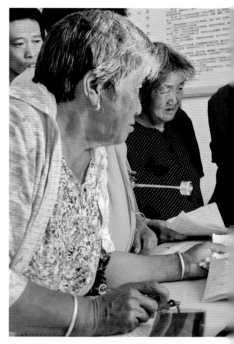

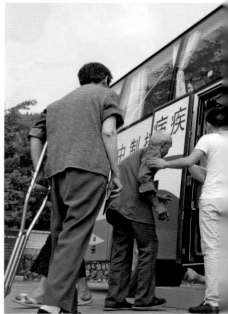

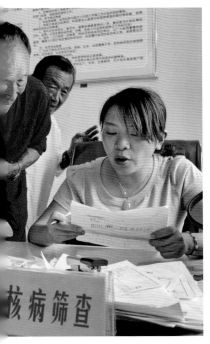

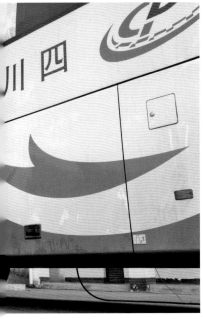

四川省江油市疾控中心在一年一度的老年人健康体检中加入了结核病筛查和结核病防治知识宣传工作。

The CDC of Jiangyou city, Sichuan includes tuberculosis screening and tuberculosis health education in the annual health checkup for the elderly.

今年的体检点就设在江油市二郎庙镇雷江村村委会。一大早这里就热闹起来了，一群穿着白大褂、带着体检设备的医生早早来到现场做准备工作。由于村里事先已发了通知，所以体检车前很快就聚集了很多老人。

The site of physical examination is located in the village council of Leijiang village, Erlangmiao township, Jiangyou. Early in the morning, a group of doctors in white coats and equipment arrived early to prepare for their work. As the villagers got the notice in advance, many elderly people gathered in front of the mobile clinic.

在老人们等待体检的过程中，工作人员上前为他们讲解结核病知识，叮嘱他们有了可疑症状赶快去医院检查等，聊着聊着就上了一堂生动的科普课。

As the elderly were waiting for the medical examination, the health workers came up to explain the TB knowledge and reminded them to go to the hospital for an examination if they had suspicious symptoms of tuberculosis. This is really like a lively science class.

当老人们从体检车出来的时候都非常高兴，说以前只能在大医院做的检查，现在在家门口就能做了，不用再折腾来折腾去，真是方便！实践充分证明，把结核病筛查工作纳入老年人健康体检是一种有效的主动发现手段。通过主动筛查，发现早期患者，及时治疗康复，降低传播风险。

After the physical examination in the mobile clinic, the elderly said that the examination previously available only in large hospitals was now done right in their neighborhood. It is much more convenient! In practice, the inclusion of tuberculosis screenings in elderly health checkups has proven to be an effective method of active detection. The risk of transmission can be reduced through active screening, early detection, timely treatment, and rehabilitation.

密切接触者筛查，减少疫情传播
CLOSE CONTACT SCREENING TO REDUCE TB EPIDEMIC

肺结核是传染性疾病，一旦发生，受累的不光是患者，还包括与其工作、生活等有过频繁密切接触的人员，这些人员都有可能受到结核菌的感染，如果不及时进行筛查，就会漏掉感染者甚至患者，他们又会成为新的传染源，造成疫情的扩散和传播。因此肺结核发生在哪里，对密切接触者的筛查就必须做到哪里。

Tuberculosis is a Infectious disease. Once being infected with TB, the patients will suffer and those who have frequent or close contact with the patients through work or social venues may also be exposed to tuberculosis. If screening is not performed in time, the infected persons or TB patients may be overlooked and they will become a new source of infection, causing the spread of the epidemic. Therefore, when cases of TB are detected, close contact screening must be done.

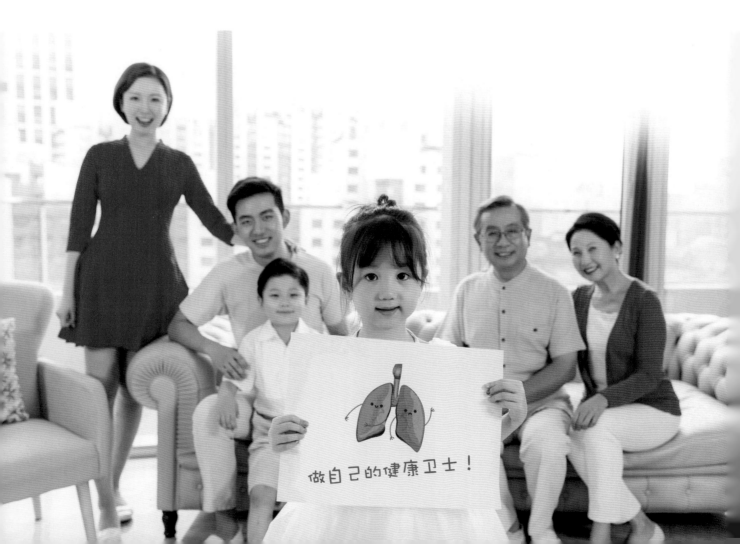

在连续两周出现咳嗽、咳痰、低热症状之后，冯先生来到县医院就诊，被诊断为肺结核。

After two weeks of cough, phlegm and fever symptoms, Mr. FENG came to the county hospital and was diagnosed with pulmonary tuberculosis.

冯先生原准备医生开具药方后就赶快取药回家，没想到医生开始详细询问他的家庭成员情况：家中有几个人？有没有老年人、未成年儿童？大家身体情况如何？有没有出现咳嗽、发热等情况？当冯先生提到自己的儿子刚刚5岁，而老母亲也有咳嗽症状后，医生要求他尽快带母亲、儿子到医院做结核病筛查，因为他们是已患病冯先生的密切接触者。

FENG had planned to get the doctor's prescription, take the medicine, and return home. But the doctor began to ask about his family members in detail: How many family members? Are there any elderly people? any children? How are they doing? Are they showing signs of cough or fever? When FENG mentioned that his son has just 5 years old and his mother had cough symptoms, the doctor asked him to bring his mother and son to the hospital for tuberculosis screenings as soon as possible, as they had close contact with FENG, an TB patient.

关系到家人的健康，冯先生不敢耽搁，第二天就带着母亲和孩子前来筛查。幸运的是，孩子身体健康，母亲的咳嗽也仅是慢性支气管炎。医生又再次向冯先生强调了诸如坚持服药、居家戴口罩、单独卧室居住、确保开窗通风、密切关注母亲和孩子健康情况等信息。冯先生一家也认识到预防结核病的重要性，认真地遵照医嘱，一项不落。

This is a matter of health for his family. FENG brought his mother and child for a screening the next day. Fortunately, the child was in good health and the mother's cough was just chronic bronchitis. The doctor once again encouraged FENG to take medicines, wear a mask at home, live in a separate bedroom, ensure ventilation by opening the windows, and pay close attention to the health of his mother and his child. FENG's family also recognized the importance of tuberculosis prevention and carefully follow the doctor's instructions.

密切接触者筛查管理
Close contact screening and management

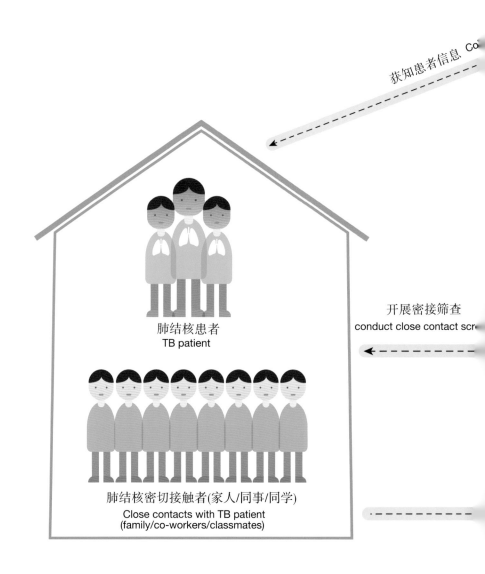

获知患者信息 Co...

肺结核患者
TB patient

开展密接筛查
conduct close contact scr...

肺结核密切接触者(家人/同事/同学)
Close contacts with TB patient
(family/co-workers/classmates)

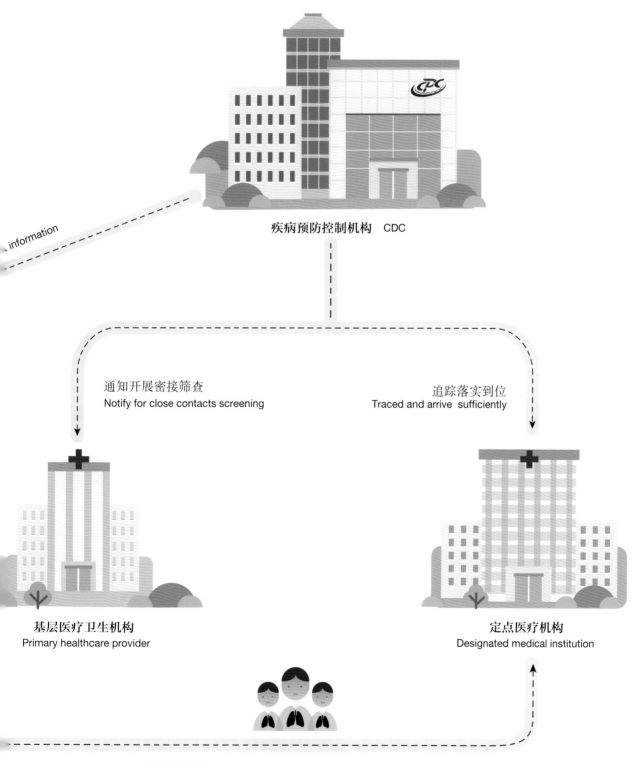

information

疾病预防控制机构　CDC

通知开展密接筛查
Notify for close contacts screening

追踪落实到位
Traced and arrive sufficiently

基层医疗卫生机构
Primary healthcare provider

定点医疗机构
Designated medical institution

有症状转诊　Transfer people with suspected TB symptom

结核菌 / 艾滋病病毒双重感染，
及时治疗就有希望

EARLY TREATMENT FOR TB/HIV
CO-INFECTION

艾滋病病毒感染者和患者免疫水平较正常人低，容易感染结核菌，这对患者来说是雪上加霜的双重打击，如果不及时治疗，会导致严重后果，甚至会危及生命。对艾滋病病毒感染者和患者，应当严格按要求进行结核病筛查，如发现有感染，应及时进行治疗。

HIV-infected people and patients have lower immune level than normal people, and are prone to TB infection, which causes.great concern. If not treated in time, it could lead to serious and even life-threatening consequences. For people living with HIV/AIDS, tuberculosis screenings should be carried out in strict accordance with the requirements. In case that an infection is found, the patient should be promptly treated.

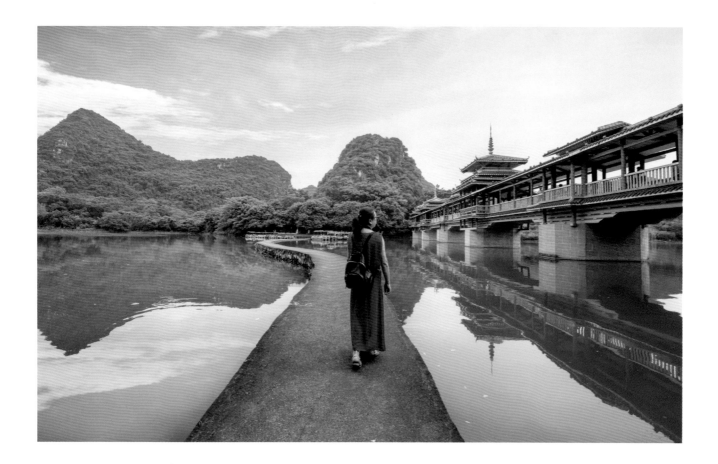

如果说疾病会使一个人的世界蒙上灰色，那么韦妹（化名）的世界曾一度是黑色的，她不仅是艾滋病病毒感染者，还是肺结核患者，她是结核菌/艾滋病病毒双重感染的患者。

If a disease may cast a shadow on one's world, then Wei Mei's world was pitch black. She was living with HIV. She was also a TB patient. She was experiencing HIV/TB co-infection.

20年前，她因肺结核大咯血窒息，在医院救治过程中同时筛查出合并艾滋病病毒感染。在她如花的年纪里，遭受如此沉重的打击让韦妹难以承受，她一度产生轻生念头，当地疾控中心工作人员一次又一次地找到她，耐心、细致地做工作，鼓励她积极治疗。在艾滋病"四免一关怀"政策和当地结核病保障政策的帮助下，韦妹撑过了漫长的黑夜等到黎明，最终治愈了肺结核，艾滋病抗病毒治疗也取得了很好的效果。

Twenty years ago, Mei was diagnosed with HIV/TB co-infection during an emergency hospital treatment for asphyxia caused by pulmonary tuberculosis-induced hemoptysis. In her blooming age, it was hard for Mei to bear such a heavy blow and she once had the idea of suicide. The local CDC staff apprached her again and again, patiently and meticulously encouraged her to seek treatment. Thanks to the "Four Frees and One Care" policy of HIV/AIDS program and the local tuberculosis care policies, Mei has survived the long, and dark night until the dawn of her tuberculosis cured. Her HIV antiretroviral treatment has also achieved good results.

如今，20年过去了，韦妹依旧健康地生活着，她感恩社会，赋予她一次新的生命。

Now, 20 years later, WEI is still living a healthy life. She is grateful to the society for giving her a new life.

第五章

智慧结控
技术创新

Chapter 5

Smart, Innovative and Forward-looking Approaches to TB Control

结核病防治的信息化建设与时俱进。

The digitization of tuberculosis prevention and control is moving ahead in step with the evolution of information technology.

以往结核病疫情报告要通过纸质"三本一表"收集信息。"三本"是初诊患者登记本、结核患者登记本和实验室登记本，"一表"是季度工作量、发现患者数和既往发现患者的治疗转归表。那时的"三本一表"所承载的就是当今信息系统的作用。

In the past, tuberculosis case reports were collected through the "three books and one sheet" method, in paper format. The "three books" constituted the registration of patients at first consultation, the registration of confirmed TB patients, and the laboratory registration. The "one sheet" was the quarterly report of workload, the number of patients detected, and the treatment outcomes of patients found in the previous period. The "three books and one sheet" played the role of today's information system.

2004年，中国开始实施传染病报告信息管理系统，开启了传染病报告信息化的先河。结防人以此为契机，于2005年建立了中国结核病管理信息系统，这一专报系统覆盖到全国所有县级防治机构，可以实时收集各地每个结核病患者诊断、治疗和转归的信息。实现了从"纸质、定时、汇总"到"电子、实时、个案"的结核病信息化飞跃式变革。同时结核病专报系统还可以与传染病网络直报系统实时进行数据交换，两个信息系统成为将综合医疗机构、结核病定点医疗机构、疾病预防控制机构间紧密联系在一起的纽带，为提高结核病患者发现、规范结核病患者归口管理、有效开展医防合作提供了信息沟通平台，成为全球结核病信息化的典范。

In 2004, China began to implement an Internet-based Infectious Disease Information System, for systematic reporting of infectious disease. Taking this opportunity, China established the Internet-based TB reporting and management system in 2005. This dedicated reporting system covers all county-level prevention and control institutions in the country and collects information in real-time on the diagnosis, treatment, and outcomes of each tuberculosis patient. This development ushered in a revolutionary change in the informatization of tuberculosis control from "paper-based, periodic aggregation" to "real-time, electronic reporting of individual cases". During this time, the dedicated tuberculosis reporting system also shares real-time data with the Infectious Disease Information System. The two information systems rally the general medical institutions, designated TB medical institutions, and CDCs around the common objectives of quickly identifying TB patients, standardizing and centralizing TB patient management, and providing effective linkages between prevention and treatment service providers. This system is regarded as model for the informatization of TB control globally.

随着"互联网+"技术的蓬勃发展，智慧结控（电子药盒、手机APP、专用平台等）、人工智能诊断、远程会诊与培训等皆在引领全球结核病患者管理新模式。

Thanks to the rapid development of *Internet plus* technologies, China is now reinventing the model of tuberculosis patient management with intelligent TB control practices (e.g. electronic medication boxes, mobile app, dedicated platforms, etc.), artificial intelligence diagnostics, and remote consultation and training.

互联网让结核病控制插上翅膀，飞得更高更远，也让结核病患者受益更多！

The internet has given TB control wings, allowing it to fly higher and further to the greater benefit of tuberculosis patients!

直报加专报信息全知道

INFECTIOUS DISEASE REPORTING SYSTEM AND TB INFORMATION MANAGEMENT SYSTEM

传染病报告信息管理系统和结核病管理信息系统的建立，是中国传染病防控历史上的里程碑。这两个系统就像传染病和结核病的"千里眼"和"顺风耳"，只要有结核病发生，我们都可以第一时间捕捉到信息，并对患者的发现、诊断、治疗和管理的全程进行密切追踪管理。

The establishment of the Infectious Disease Reporting System and TB Information Management System was a milestone in the history of infectious disease prevention and control in China. Both systems act as the eyes and ears on the ground for monitoring infectious diseases and tuberculosis. We can capture information as soon as new cases of tuberculosis occurs and closely track the patients throughout diagnosis, treatment, and follow-up management.

赵医生在市疾控中心结防科工作，一大早他跟往常一样熟练地打开电脑进入传染病报告信息管理系统和结核病管理信息系统浏览信息。突然，一个就诊于外省胸科医院的肺结核患者跃入他的眼帘。此患者为一名13岁的儿童，赵医生马上进行信息核实，并立即把患者情况报告至省疾控中心，一场跨省的沟通就此展开，最终核明了患者的情况。这就是传染病直报+结核病专报两大信息系统的协同作用，为第一时间追踪结核病患者，之后尽快展开诊断、治疗和管理工作奠定了坚实的基础。

Dr. ZHAO works at the tuberculosis control department of the local CDC. Early in the morning, he turned on his computer and logged into the two information systems, as he did most days. Suddenly, a tuberculosis patient receiving treatment at a chest hospital outside the province caught his eyes. The patient was only 13 years old. Dr. ZHAO immediately checked the information and reported the case to the provincial CDC, where cross-provincial communication began to verify the patient's condition. This is an example of the synergy between the two information systems, which provide a solid foundation for tracking TB patients as they are reported in addition to monitoring their diagnosis, treatment, and management as expeditiously as possible.

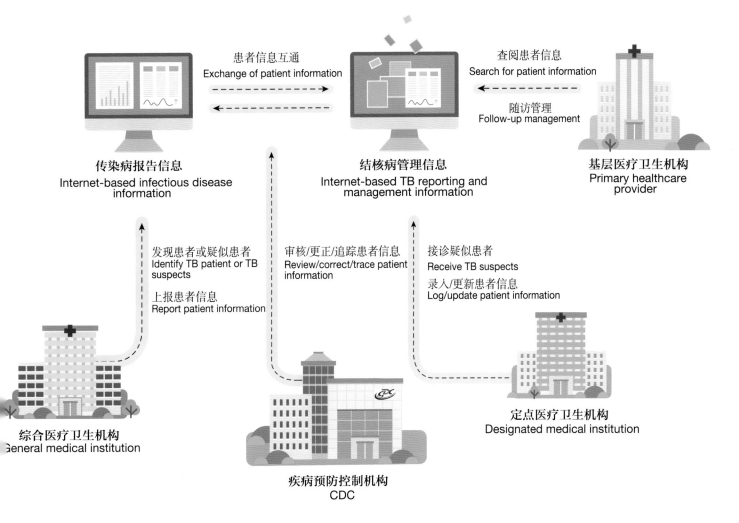

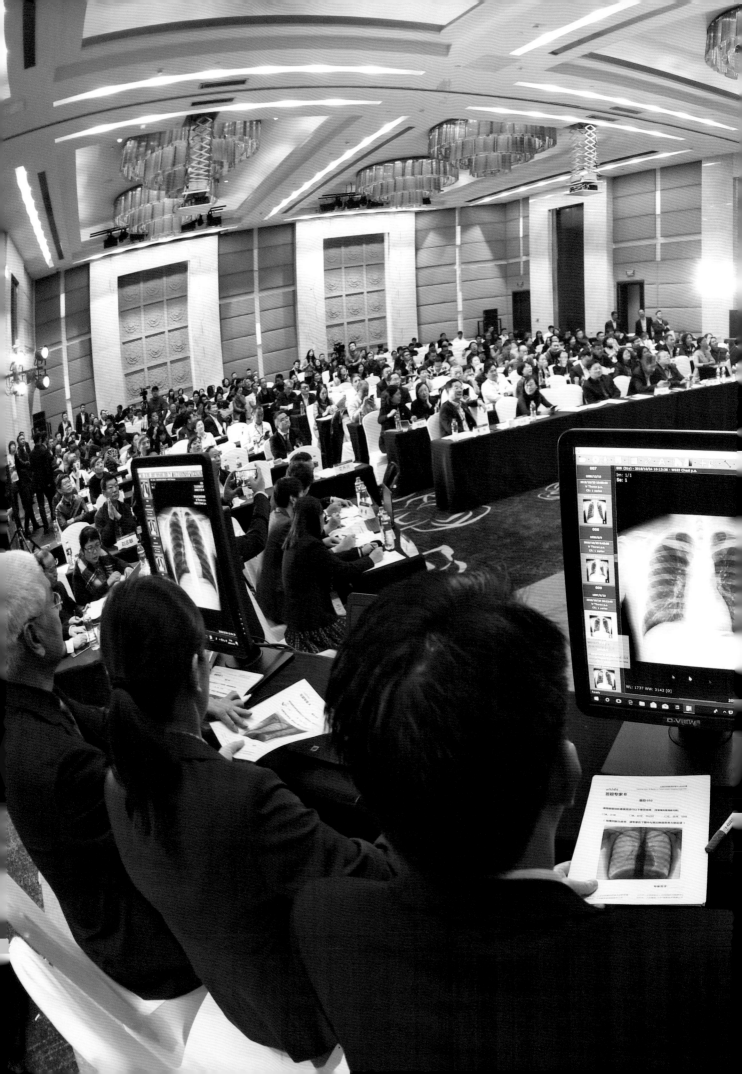

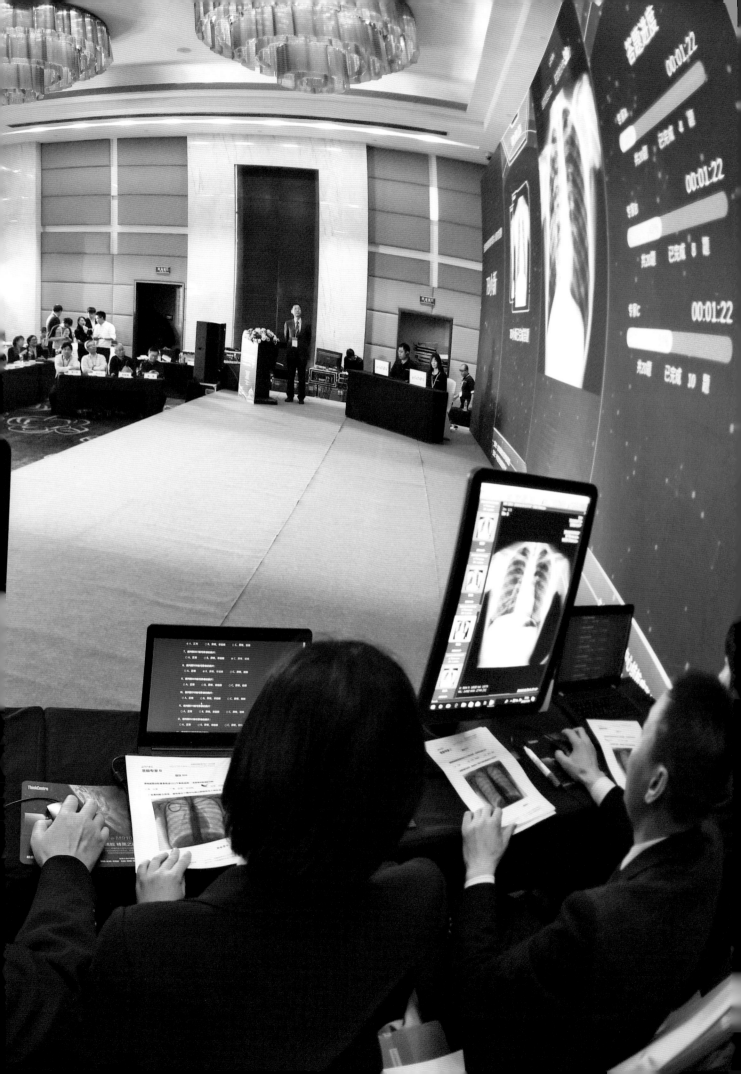

人工智能技术助力结核病诊断
ARTIFICIAL INTELLIGENCE FACILITATING TB DIAGNOSIS

在速度体现效率与生命的时代，结核病的诊断也搭上高速发展的智能之车。惊心动魄的人机大战，不仅仅是专家和机器阅读胸片时间与质量的较量，更有意义的是，这将会为结核病患者赢得更及时的治疗时间，获得更显著的成本效益。

In a time when speed is critical, TB diagnosis also undergoes rapid development. The thrilling human-machine collaboration is not only one of radiologists and machines interpreting the chest radiographs with the least time and best accuracy; more meaningfully, human-machine cooperation allows TB patients more timely access to treatment and helps the health system achieve greater cost-effectiveness.

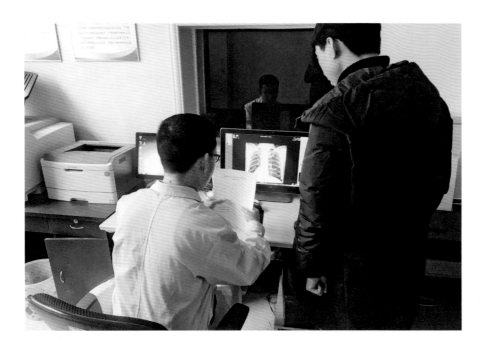

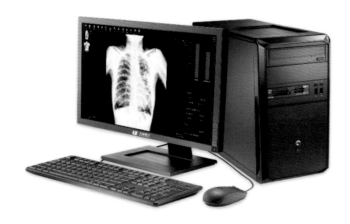

肺结核智能筛查工作站
TB smart screening workstation

张家口市怀来县（河北）卫生院的陈医生一大早就来到了办公室，今天是医院配备的肺结核智能筛查工作站验收的日子。这项技术已经获得了国家食品药品监督管理总局（CFDA）认证，使肺结核诊断更加经济高效，将有望在中低收入地区疾病防控和健康扶贫工作中开展应用。

Dr. CHEN from Huailai county township hospital in Zhangjiakou city (Hebei) came into the office early this morning. This was the first day his hospital would be equipped with the new tuberculosis intelligent screening workstation. This technology was certified by the State Food and Drug Administration (CFDA), making pulmenary tuberculosis diagnosis more cost-effective. The new workstation was expected to be used to tackle disease prevention for poverty alleviation in low- and middle-income areas.

此智能筛查工作站是以人工智能（AI）算法为基础，用大量的肺结核影像样本及专家标注数据进行深度学习，以图形处理单元（GPU）云计算为平台开发出的一套结核病诊断系统。工作站利用人工智能技术高速且精准的技术特性，对结核病患者的影像资料进行智能筛查，发现符合肺结核的影像特征后直接发出疾病辅助诊断提示，可以帮助医生快速完成精准的诊断过程，减少人工诊断出现的漏诊和误诊，提升诊断质量。

This intelligent screening workstation is a tuberculosis diagnostic system based on artificial intelligence (AI) algorithms. It uses a large number of pulmonary tuberculosis radiograph samples and expert labeling data for deep learning, and it operates on a cloud platform powered by graphic processing units (GPUs). Leveraging the speed and precision that comes with artificial intelligence technology, the workstation performs intelligent screening of a TB patient's image data, compares it against known image profiles of TB, and then directly generates auxiliary diagnosis remarks. This workstation is a great tool for doctors to quickly complete an accurate diagnosis process, reduce possible omission and misdiagnosis by human radiologists, and improve the reliability of diagnoses.

以一位医生查阅一个患者的胸片花费3分钟来计算，一位影像科医生一天能够查看160例患者的胸片。而在AI读片机器人"TB小新"的辅助下，影像筛查的时间可以缩短到2秒钟，一天就能够查阅近15 000例患者的影像，筛查效率大幅度提升，特别是在体检、流行病学调查、初筛工作中更能大显身手！

A physician spends 3 minutes on each patient's chest radiograph, and can view 160 patients' chest radiographs a day. But with the aid of the AI radiology robot "TB Xiaoxin", the time for image screening can be shortened to 2 seconds, and the images of nearly 15,000 patients can be reviewed one day – a significant improvement in screening productivity. This is especially useful in physical examination, epidemiological investigation, and initial screening!

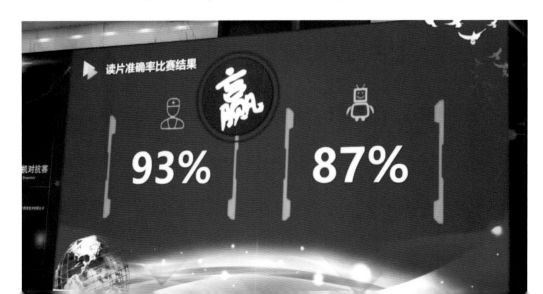

结核病影像读片"人机大战"中，"TB小新"与专家的准确率几乎平分秋色
In the human vs. machine competition for TB image review, TB Xiaoxin nearly matches the expert radiologist's accuracy.

智慧结控助力患者管理

SMART TUBERCULOSIS CONTROL LEADING TO BETTER PATIENT MANAGEMENT

中国互联网+医疗健康战略的春风正在吹向结核病防控管理工作的创新发展，即便在广大的偏远地区，也阻隔不了智能远程诊疗技术带给患者的福音，医务人员和患者的随访距离不再需用脚步丈量，而替代为数据线的连接与智能电子药盒等实时传递的信息，这些变化带来的是广覆盖、更省时、更高效、更精准的防治管理服务。

China's Internet + Medical Health Strategy is driving innovation and progress in tuberculosis prevention and control. The benefits of smart, remote diagnostic and treatment solutions trickle down to patients in remote areas. In follow-up activities, the distance between medical personnel and patients no longer needs to be measured in footsteps, instead by real-time information transmitted via data cables from smart electronic medicine boxes. These changes bring about expansive coverage, time savings, productivity gains, and better targeted prevention and control services.

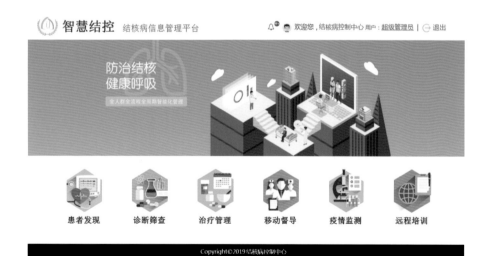

智慧结控

Intelligent Tuberculosis Control

一部手机、一款应用，一端连接患者，一端连接医疗机构。"智慧结控"就像一个全天候的私人健康管家。

The mobile phone app, "Intelligent Tuberculosis Control", that connects patients and health providers serves as a 24/7 personal health butler.

一个叫谢纯（化名）的年轻人在深圳市南山区被诊断为肺结核，在接受规范治疗时，除了常规到医院取药、复查，通过"智慧结控"微信小程序，每天录制服药视频上传至客户端，社区医生可及时掌握他的服药情况和病情变化，若忘记服药或发生不良反应，在线医务人员就会立即通过语音、视频及时提醒并给予帮助，出现药物不良反应还可以留言或联系医生及时指导和处理。

A young man named XIE Chun was diagnosed with pulmonary tuberculosis in Nanshan district, Shenzhe and received the standard treatment. In addition to routine visits to the hospital to pick up his medicine and undergo follow-up examinations, he also used a WeChat mini-program called "Intelligent Tuberculosis Control" to record his daily medicine taking and to upload the video through the program. The community doctor can then track his adherence and possible changes to his condition. If the patient forgot to take his medicine or had an adverse reaction, the online medical staff would immediately intervene with instructions or assistance by voice or video. In case of an adverse reaction, the patient can send a message or contact a doctor for further intervention.

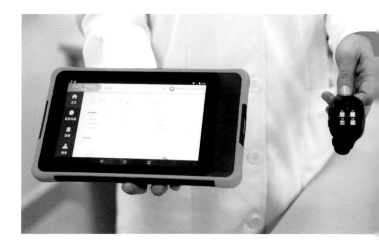

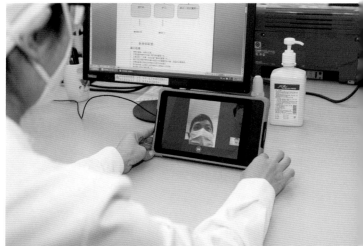

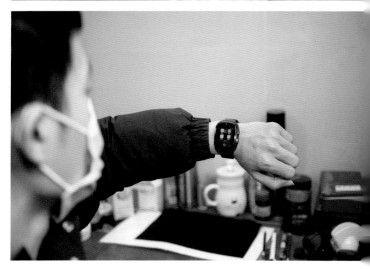

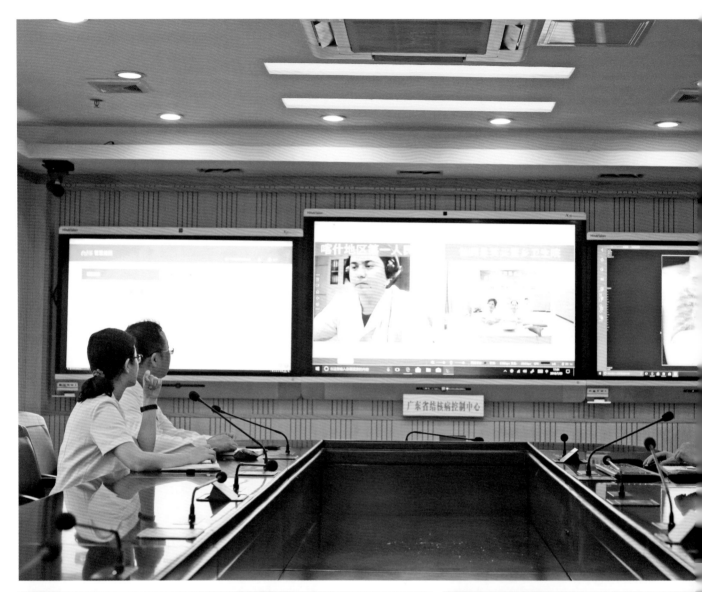

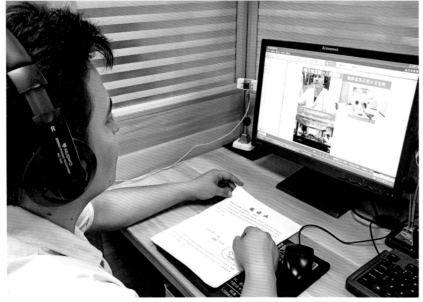

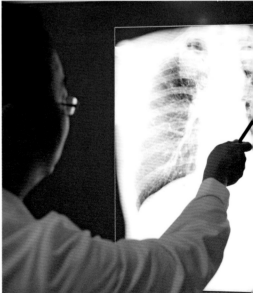

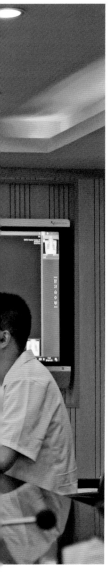

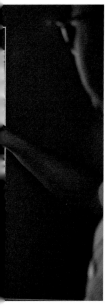

"智慧结控"还将精准扶贫的纽带延伸至新疆喀什地区，建设一条结核病防治的"信息化高速公路"，连接边疆地区的定点医院、疾控中心和乡镇卫生院，打破信息壁垒，让医疗数据"动起来"。为解决边疆地区基层医生影像诊断水平相对薄弱的问题，"智慧结控"搭建了结核病云影像和远程诊疗平台，人工智能诊断最快能在10分钟内完成诊断评价，显著减少患者延误诊断的情况。远在千里之外的专家还可通过结核病快速远程影像传输及会诊的方式，为边疆的疑难病例作诊断指导。

"Intelligent Tuberculosis Control" also extends the reach of targeted poverty alleviation to the Kashgar region in Xinjiang. The program creates an "information superhighway" for tuberculosis prevention and control, connecting to designated hospitals, CDCs, and rural health centers in border areas and breaking down information barriers to facilitate the flow of medical data. Recognizing that primary care physicians in the frontier areas have low capacity for radiograph reading, the "Intelligent Tuberculosis Control" cloud-based imaging and remote diagnosis platform has been established. The AI assistant can complete diagnoses and evaluations in as short as 10 minutes, and significantly reducing delays in diagnosis. Specialists a thousand miles away can provide guidance for difficult and complex cases in the frontier areas by means of rapid remote transmission of images and joint consultation.

"智慧结控"搭建的结核病云影像和远程诊疗平台
TB cloud imaging and remote diagnostic and treatment platform built as part of Intelligent Tuberculosis Control

数据跑路代替医生跑腿

Data travels instead of doctors

徐伦斌在贵州省清镇市站街镇卫生院工作了很多年，他说以前结核病患者随访资料都是手工填写，总是担心出错，贵州属边远山区，交通不发达，所以每次报送都要花费很长时间。但现在好了，清镇建成了全省首个覆盖全市区域的基层结核病患者健康管理平台—"卫计通"APP。全市14个乡镇300多个村医自从用上这款"卫计通"后，每次随访治疗管理只要带一部手机就可以了，而且还能够实现管理信息秒报回传，真的让"数据跑路"代替了"医生跑腿"，关键是准确且有效率，极大地方便了患者。

XU Lunbin worked for many years at the Zhenjie tonwnship hospital in Qingzhen city, Guizhou province. He said that previously the follow-up data of tuberculosis patients was filled out by hand, and that he was always worried about errors. Guizhou is a remote mountainous area with underdeveloped traffic, so it takes a long time to submit reach report. Now, the situation has improved dramatically. Qingzhen is now the first in Guizhou to use the app "Health Connection" (Wei Ji Tong pronounced in Chinese). It is a health management platform for all the tuberculosis patients in the city.

More than 300 village doctors in 14 townships across the city can use Health Connection, allowing them to perform follow-up and manage patients using just a mobile phone. Doctors can also send and receive patient information in seconds. This is a paradigm shift from "traveling doctors" to "traveling data". More importantly, the accuracy and efficiency gains benefit patients.

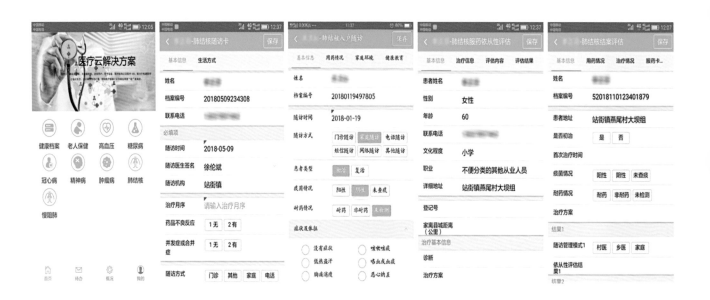

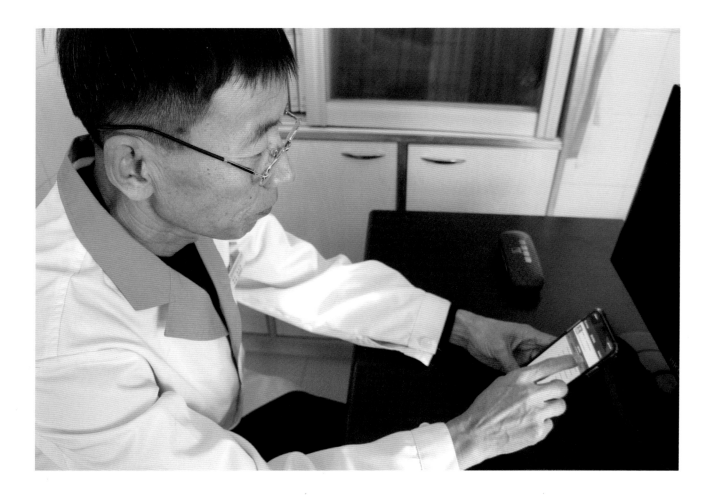

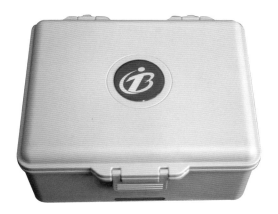

电子药盒等智能工具为肺结核患者带来福音

Smart tools, such as electronic medicine boxes, bring good news to tuberculosis patients

61岁的肺结核患者李老汉家距离村卫生室有5公里，他孤身一人没人督促服药，定点医院的医生和村医商量后决定给他使用电子智能药盒。

LI, a 61-year-old, male tuberculosis patient, lives 5 kilometers away from the village clinic. He lives alone so no one supervises his medicine taking. After a brief discussion, the doctors at the designated hospital and the village clinic decided to give him a smart electronic medicine box.

每天7点早饭前，智能药盒会提醒李老汉服药，他打开智能药盒，取出药品，按时服药，将剩余药品放回去，再关闭智能药盒，这一系列动作都会被完整记录下来。与此同时，村医会打开与智能药盒相连的手机APP，查看他的服药情况。有一天，已经10点了，村医发现他还没服药，赶快打电话问明情况，原来李老汉早上6点有急事要出门就没来得及吃，村医督促他回去后一定要马上服药，下午手机APP提示李老汉已经完成服药了。智能药盒既是李老汉贴心的"助手"，也是他的毫不留情的"监督员"，在智能药盒的帮助下，李老汉全程规范治疗，治愈了肺结核，他高兴地把电子药盒归还给了村医！

The smart medicine box could remind LI to take his medicine every day at 7 AM, before breakfast. The entire series of actions could be recorded, when he opened the box to take out the right pills, put the remaining pills back, and closed the box.. The village doctor would open a mobile app corresponding to the smart medicine box to check LI's adherence. One

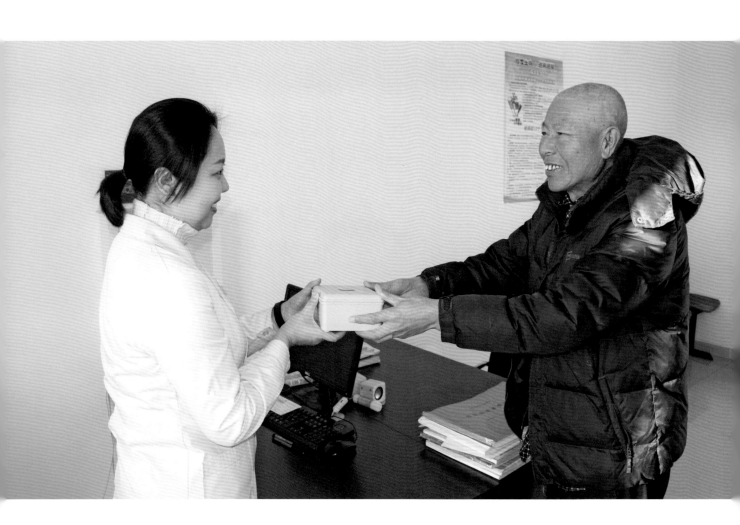

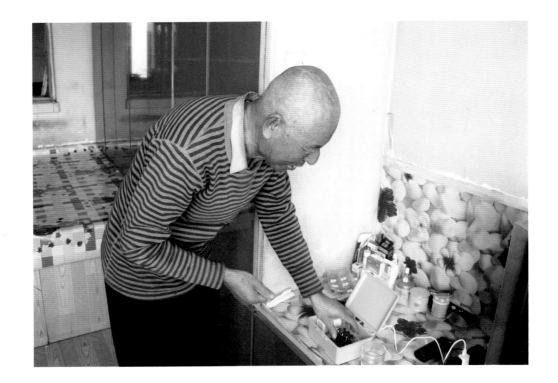

day after 10 AM, the village doctor found that LI had not taken his medicine and called him. It turned out that LI had to leave in a hurry at 6 AM for some emergency, so he did not take his medicine. The village doctor urged him to take the medicine as soon as he returned home. In the afternoon, the mobile phone app indicated that LI had finally taken his medicine. The smart medicine box is both a thoughtful "assistant" to LI and a strict "supervisor". With the help of the smart kit, LI completed the standard treatment, cured his tuberculosis, and happily returned the electronic medicine box to the village doctor!

采用电子智能药盒和手机技术，在不同地理条件、经济状况下对肺结核患者进行治疗管理，不仅方便患者和医务人员，降低成本，还可显著提高患者治疗的依从性，帮助患者完成规范治疗的全过程。

The use of electronic smart kit and mobile phone technologies to manage tuberculosis patients in challenging geographic and economic conditions not only makes it easier for patients and medical personnel, but also significantly improves patient compliance and completion of the entire standard treatment.

远程培训学习永无止境

CONSTANT CAPACITY BUILDING BY REMOTE TRAINING

借助互联网技术，中国结核病远程医疗咨询与培训平台服务正在各级结核病诊疗机构、尤其是基层医疗卫生服务机构广泛开展，基层工作者足不出户就能及时获得最新知识的学习，这对提升基层防治人员的业务水平起到了无可替代的作用。能力建设也插上互联网的翅膀向着更高、更远的方向飞去！

With the help of the internet technology, China's tuberculosis telemedicine consultation and training platforms are used at the various levels of healthcare providers for tuberculosis diagnosis and treatment, especially primary healthcare institutions. The grass-roots health workers can acquire the latest knowledge without leaving office, and they can better provide high-quality services with improved capacity and updated information. Thanks to the internet technology, capacity building is now accessible in even the most remote areas.

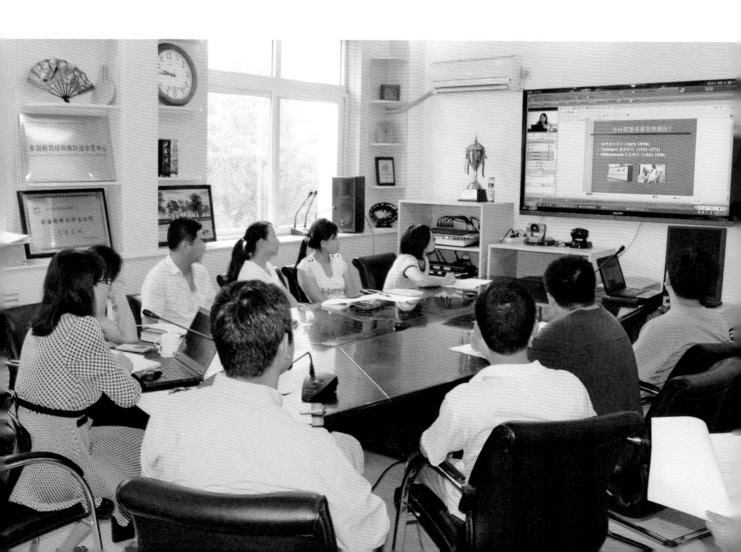

中国西部某市肺科医院的小范医生忙完上午的门诊，很快就被通知下午要参加一次学习。小范之前就知道了今天的学习内容，他很期待，因为讲课的是国家级的结核病专家，能够听到这样的课对于西部地区的基层工作者真是太难得了！关键是不仅可以听课，还可以与专家进行互动答疑，解决平时工作中遇到的疑难问题，与同行在线交流学习。

Dr. FAN from a lung hospital in western China just completed his outpatient shift for the morning and was asked to attend a training session in the afternoon. Dr. FAN knew about the training and was looking forward to it because the lecturer was given by a respected TB expert in the country. It was hard for Dr. FAN and the other primary healthcare workers in western China to get a chance for such a lecture and, even more encouraging that they could interact with the expert on line to answer their queries.

如今，远程平台的便捷性、在时间和地点上的灵活性、长期可持续性、经济性等优势逐渐显现，受到基层结核病医院和医生的欢迎，加入远程平台的单位也越来越多。截至2019年底，全国已有243家结核病诊疗机构加入远程平台。远程活动的内容和形式也在不断更新和完善，邀请国内外著名专家授课、为西藏自治区和新疆维吾尔自治区量身定制远程培训计划、支持各种病例讨论等。

Nowadays, the advantages of the telemedicine platforms are increasingly recognized such as easy access, flexibility in time and place, long-term sustainability, and economy, widely adopted by primary tuberculosis hospitals and doctors. At the end of 2019, 243 TB clinics had adopted telemedicine platforms, and the content and forms of remote activities are constantly updated and improved. Such activities include the lectures given by the renowned Chinese and international experts, tailored remote training programs for the health workers in Tibet and Xinjiang autonomous regions, and case-study based discussions on tuberculosis.

第六章

国际合作
发展共赢

Chapter 6

International
Cooperation
for Common
Development

中国始终以开放的姿态拥抱全世界。结核病防治一直以来都是全球化课题，中国秉持"引进来，走出去"的国际合作理念对全球共同消灭结核病发挥着积极的作用。

China has always embraced the world with an open mind. Recognizing that tuberculosis is a global challenge, China has adhered to the "bringing in, going global" philosophy of international engagement. This philosophy has played a positive role in shaping global efforts to end tuberculosis.

中国政府与国际伙伴建立了广泛而深入的合作关系。如世界银行，英国国际发展署、抗击艾滋病、结核病和疟疾全球基金，比尔及梅琳达·盖茨基金会，世界卫生组织，比利时达米恩基金会，美国疾病控制与预防中心，梅里埃基金会等，呈现出合作伙伴多、资金量大、覆盖面广、业务领域宽、持续时间长的特点，不仅为中国结核病防治工作提供了大量的资金、技术和先进的防治理念，也通过项目的实施，培养和锻炼了一批结核病防治骨干。

The Chinese government has established close and extensive partnerships with international partners such as the World Bank, UK Department for International Development, Global Fund to Fight AIDS, Tuberculosis and Malaria, Bill & Melinda Gates Foundation, World Health Organization, Damien Foundation Belgium, US Centers for Disease Control and Prevention, and Merière Foundation. The generous grants, wide coverage, scope of program activities, and long duration of support from partners has provided funds, technologies, and advanced prevention and control methods to China in addition to having developed and trained a large workforce of tuberculosis prevention and control.

在与结核病长期斗争的过程中，中国积累了符合自己国情的经验和模式：中国的结核病控制策略、医防结合模式、结核病管理信息系统和结核病防治规划评估方法等，都已成为国际推崇和学习的典范。《新英格兰医学杂志》《柳叶刀》等顶级医学期刊上有中国结核病防治的科学研究成果。全面、系统地宣传中国结核病防治工作成就的英文版《现代中国结核病控制：成就与挑战》一书，获得国际赞誉。

During its prolonged battle against tuberculosis, China has accumulated a number of experiences and models that cater to its own national conditions. China's tuberculosis prevention and control strategy, integrated model of medicine and prevention, TB information system, and TB control planning and evaluation method have become a source of inspiration and learning for its international counterparts. Top medical journals such as the New England Journal of Medicine and Lancet have featured scientific the research on tuberculosis control in China. The English edition of the book, *Tuberculosis Control in Modern China: Achievements and Challenges*, which provides a clear and systematic picture of China's achievements on tuberculosis prevention and control, has received international acclaim.

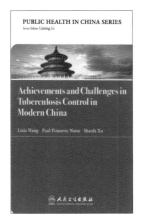 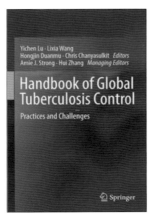 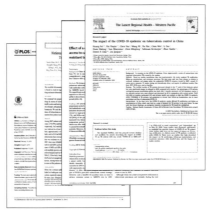 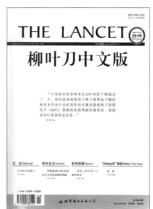

中国结核病专家在世界卫生组织、国际防痨联盟等国际组织担任重要职务，国际结核病防治舞台上有中国声音和中国观点，国际结核病防治指南里有中国的研究成果和中国专家的贡献。中国结防人为世界结核病防治工作所做出的成绩与贡献受到了国际社会的认可，获得多项国际嘉奖。

Chinese TB experts are also taking up important positions in international organizations such as the World Health Organization (WHO) and the International Union Against Tuberculosis and Lung Disease. Chinese voices and views are present on the international stage of TB control. The research findings and submissions of Chinese tuberculosis experts have been included in the *WHO Guidelines on Tuberculosis Infection Prevention and Control*. The achievements and contributions by the Chinese TB control community have been recognized by the international community and received numerous international awards.

近年来，随着综合国力提升、国际地位提高，中国正加大"走出去"的力度，迈向世界舞台，如共同搭建互通互联的中、日、韩合作交流和中亚交流互访平台，增进亚太地区结核病防控工作；发起的结核病防治援外项目，面向非洲、中亚、"一带一路"24个国家和地区开展培训和交流工作。

In recent years, with growing strength and international status, China is stepping up its efforts to "go global" and come onto the world stage. These efforts include the joint establishment of an inter-connectivity platform among China, Japan, and South Korea and the mutual exchange and visit program with Central Asia to promote progress on tuberculosis prevention and control in the Asia-Pacific region. Additionally, China has launched foreign aid training and exchange programs for TB prevention and control, targeting Africa, Central Asia, and some 24 countries and regions along the Belt and Road Initiative.

传染病无国界，终止结核病流行需要全球共同努力，在构建人类命运共同体的今天，实现无结核病的中国、无结核病的世界，需要我们和全球一道，携起手来，共同努力！

There is no national boundaries for the spread of infectious diseases. Ending tuberculosis requires a global effort. Today, to build a Community of Shared Future for Mankind and to achieve a tuberculosis-free China and world, we must join hands and work together as one united international community!

国际合作，因结核而结合

SOLIDARITY OF UNITE INTERNATIONAL PARTNERS IN THE FIGHT AGAINST TB

结核病是中国面临的严峻公共卫生问题，为了解决这个问题，自2001年以来，中国以结核病防治规划为先导，有序引进一批国际合作项目，科学统筹国内外资源，充分发挥国际项目优势，逐步摸索出了一条具有中国特色的国际合作策略。

Tuberculosis is a serious public health challenge in China. Starting in 2001, China implemented a national tuberculosis prevention and control program to introduce a pipeline of international projects in an orderly manner, sensibly aligned domestic and international resources, and fully leveraged the comparative strengths of international partners. In this process, China gradually defined a strategy for international cooperation with Chinese characteristics.

通过引进世界银行贷款/英国赠款中国结核病控制项目、全球基金中国结核病控制项目、中国国家卫生健康委员会–盖茨基金会结核病防治合作项目和世界卫生组织结核病控制项目等国际合作项目，为部分地区肺结核可疑症状者和患者的早期发现、诊断、治疗和管理，质量监控，人员能力建设，健康教育和创新研究等提供了经费和技术支持。

Through the World Bank/DFID Tuberculosis Control Project, the Global Fund China Tuberculosis Control Project, the China National Health Commission-Bill and Melinda Gates Foundation Tuberculosis Prevention and Control Project, and the World Health Organization Tuberculosis Control Project, among others, China has channeled international funding and technical supporting for the early detection, diagnosis, treatment, and management of TB cases in some locales, as well as for quality control, capacity building, health education, and innovative research.

通过探索汲取了以下经验：以规划为主导的项目设计理念，围绕规划的目标及各项措施而进行设计；建立了以政府投入为主、多方合作的筹资模式，最大限度地发挥各个项目的优势，支持中国的结核病防治规划；实施了与国际项目联合督导的方法，减少项目各自督导对基层产生的负担，同时又充分发挥各自项目专家的作用；引入了先进的项目管理理念，包括技术管理、经费管理和质量管理，提升了规划和项目的实施水平；探索了新的防治模式和策略，通过项目探索了流动人口、结核菌/艾滋病病毒双重感染和耐多药结核病等的防治模式，同时利用全球最新的技术，发展了中国的结核病控制策略。

Through experimentation, China has gained the following experiences: planning-led program design concepts, to conduct design around the planning objectives and measures; the establishment of a fundraising model with government as the primary funding source and other stakeholders as supplementary sources, to maximize the strengths of each project in support of China's tuberculosis prevention and control plans; the implementation of annual joint supervision mission with all international partners, to reduce the burden of the grass-roots health workers caused by the decentralized supervision of the different programs; the introduction of advanced project management practices, including technical management, financial management, and quality management to improve the final deliverables of the National TB prevention and control program; the exploration the creative models and strategies of TB prevention and control such as the prevention and control of tuberculosis among the migrant population, HIV/TB co-infection, and multidrug-resistant tuberculosis, and the use of state-of-the-art technologies to inform and advance China's tuberculosis control strategy.

在国际项目的支持下，中国结核病防治队伍建设和能力水平取得明显提升，推动了现代结核病控制策略（DOTS）的全面实施，促进了患者发现和治疗的效果，为全球结核病防控贡献了中国经验。

With the support of international projects, China has witnessed significant improvements in the capacity and skills of the TB control workforce, which has also fully promoted the implementation of TB control strategies including DOTS strategy, as well as the improved patient detection and treatment outcomes and connected Chinese experiences to global efforts against tuberculosis.

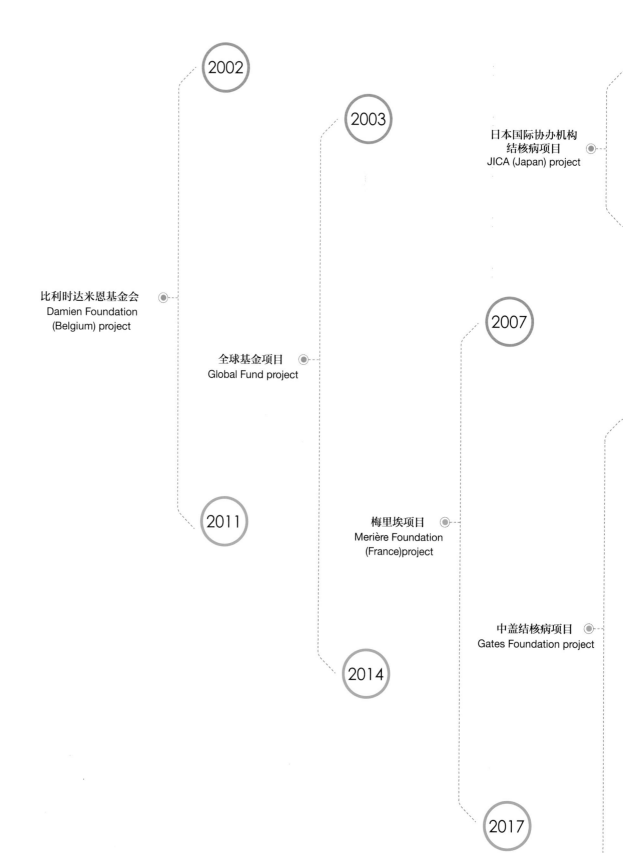

2002

2003

日本国际协办机构
结核病项目
JICA (Japan) project

比利时达米恩基金会
Damien Foundation
(Belgium) project

全球基金项目
Global Fund project

2007

2011

梅里埃项目
Merière Foundation
(France)project

2014

中盖结核病项目
Gates Foundation project

2017

结核病国际合作项目
Tuberculosis international coorperation progamme

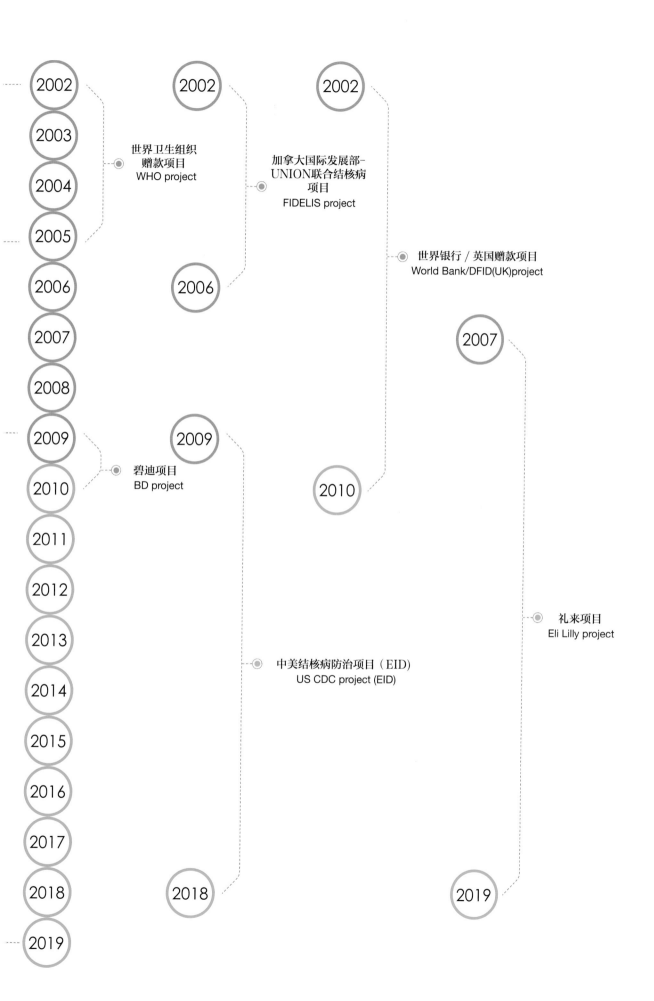

2002

2003

2004

2005

2006

2007

2008

2009

2010

2011

2012

2013

2014

2015

2016

2017

2018

2019

2002

2006

2009

2018

2002

2010

2007

2019

世界卫生组织
赠款项目
WHO project

加拿大国际发展部-
UNION联合结核病
项目
FIDELIS project

世界银行／英国赠款项目
World Bank/DFID(UK)project

碧迪项目
BD project

中美结核病防治项目（EID)
US CDC project (EID)

礼来项目
Eli Lilly project

国际舞台，发出中国声音

CHINA'S VOICE HEARD ON THE INTERNATIONAL STAGE

中国政府广泛开展多边、双边的国际交流与合作。多年来，中国专家积极参加世界卫生大会、世界卫生组织西太平洋区域委员会会议、世界肺部健康大会、金砖国家峰会、G20高峰论坛等国际会议，与世界各国交流结核病防治进展，分享中国结核病的成功经验。特别是2017年召开的第一届世界卫生组织终止结核病全球部长级会议和2018年召开的联合国大会防治结核病问题高级别会议，中国国家卫生健康委员会领导做大会报告，传播中国经验，贡献中国力量。

The Chinese government has conducted extensive multilateral and bilateral exchanges and cooperation. Over the years, Chinese experts have actively participated in international conferences such as the World Health Assembly, the World Health Organization's Western Pacific Regional Assembly, the Union World Conference on Lung Health, BRICS summits, and G20 summits to share China's progress of TB prevention and control and best practices with other countries. In particular, leaders of the National Health Commission of China presented at the first World Health Organization Global Ministerial Conference on Ending TB in 2017 and at the United Nations High-Level Meeting on Tuberculosis in 2018 to spread China's experience and show China's strength.

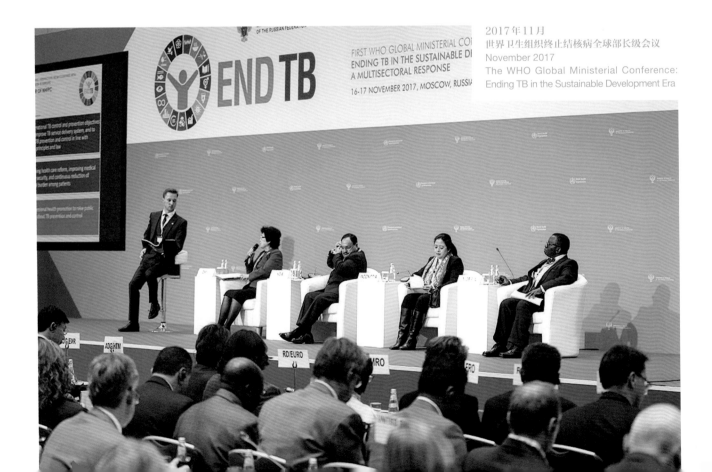

2017年11月
世界卫生组织终止结核病全球部长级会议
November 2017
The WHO Global Ministerial Conference:
Ending TB in the Sustainable Development Era

2018年7月
第八届金砖国家卫生部长会议
July 2018
The 8th BRICS Health Ministers Meeting

2018年10月
世界肺部健康大会
October 2018
The 49th World Conference on Lung Health

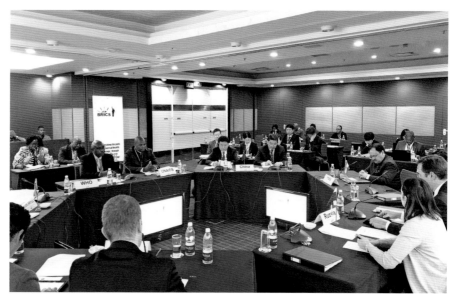

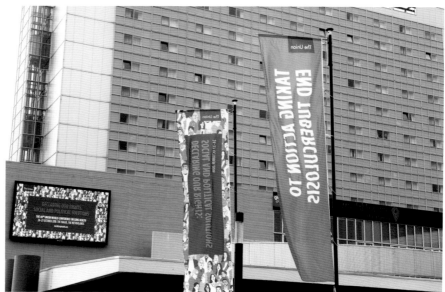

在2017年签署的金砖国家领导人厦门宣言中，中国提出建立金砖国家结核病研究网络的倡议，为金砖五国结核病研究合作提供了平台。2018年，由中国牵头起草了APEC终止结核病流行合作框架，在亚太经济合作组织第26次领导人非正式会议上讨论通过。还多次在世界肺部健康大会上举办了中国专场交流。中国正由以往的接受援助、吸收经验向加大对外援助、向外传播经验转变，中国声音正在结核病防治领域不断走向世界！

In 2017 Xiamen Declaration of BRICS Leaders, China proposed the initiative to establish the BRICS TB Research Network as a platform for cooperation in tuberculosis study among the five BRICS members. In 2018, China spearheaded the drafting of the APEC End Tuberculosis Collaboration Framework, which was discussed and endorsed at the 26th APEC Informal Leaders' Meeting. China also hosted multiple special sessions at the World Conference on Lung Health. China is increasingly shifting its role from a recipient of aid and expertise to a provider of aid and best practices to the rest of the world. The Chinese voice is increasingly vocal on the world stage in the field of tuberculosis prevention and control.

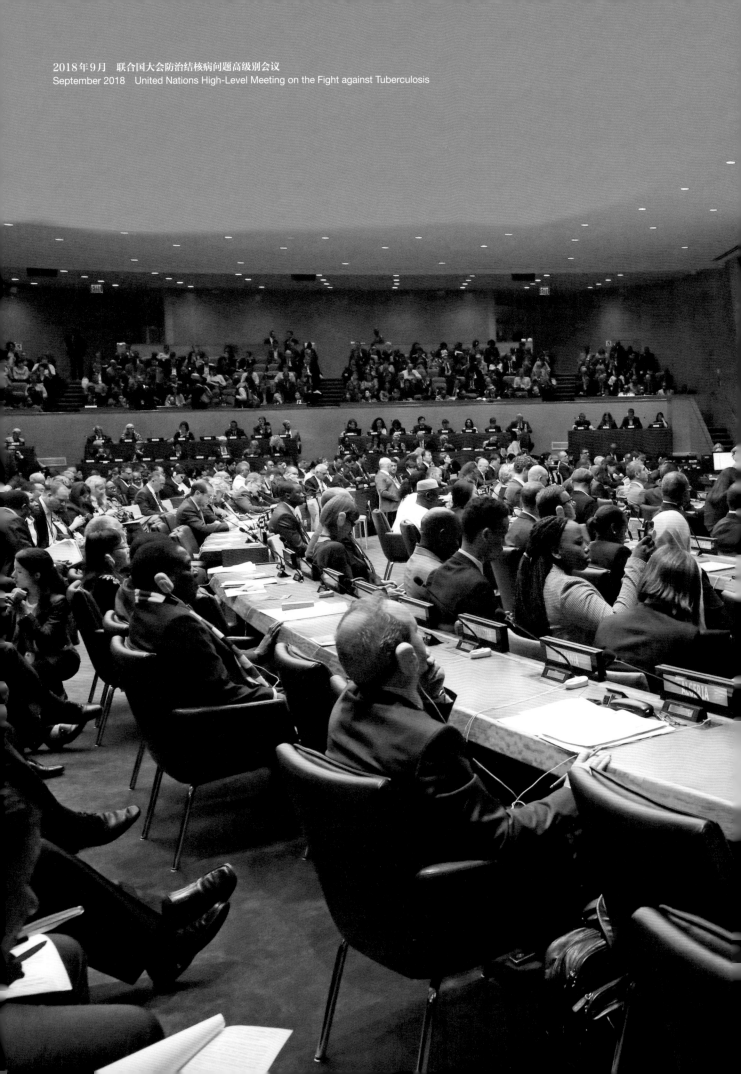

2018年9月　联合国大会防治结核病问题高级别会议
September 2018　United Nations High-Level Meeting on the Fight against Tuberculosis

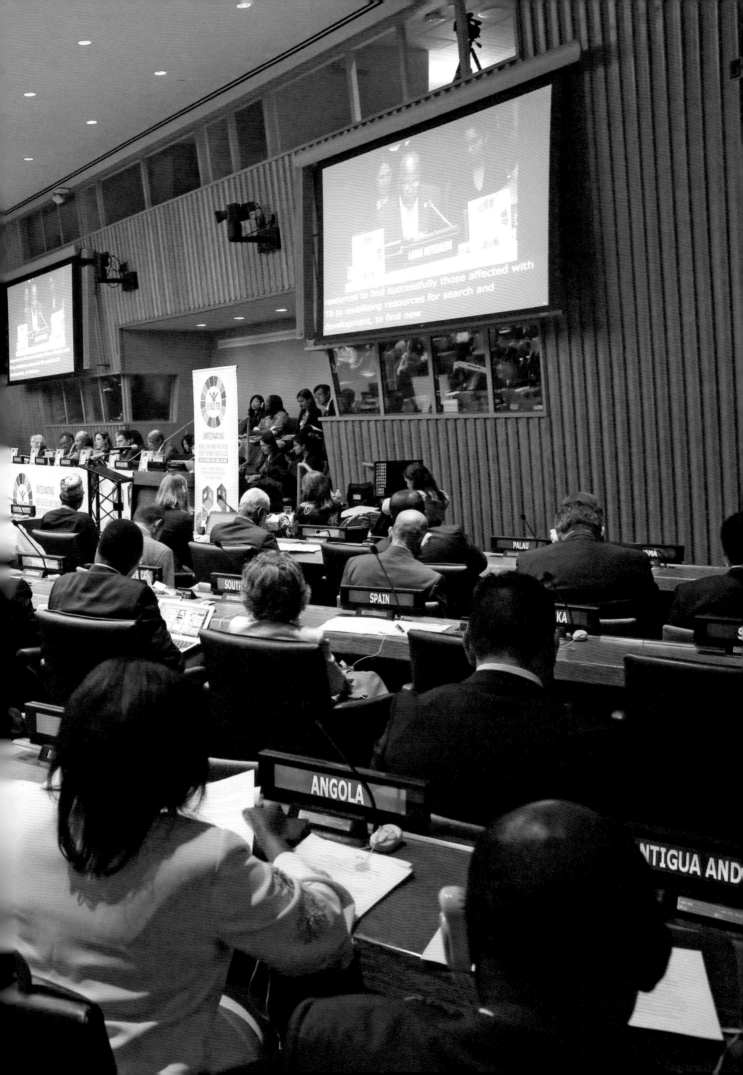

国际交流，分享中国经验
CHINA'S PRACTICES SHARED THROUGH INTERNATIONAL ENGAGEMENT

在抗击结核病方面，中国一直秉持"开放共赢"的态度，不断开展结核病防治对外交流，同时积极开展对外援助人员培训工作，培训覆盖东亚、中亚、东南亚乃至非洲等多个国家和地区。

In the fight against tuberculosis, China has always adopted an "open and win-win" approach to pursue international exchange on TB prevention and control. It continues to train foreign aid workers, covering many regions such as East Asia, Central Asia, Southeast Asia, and Africa.

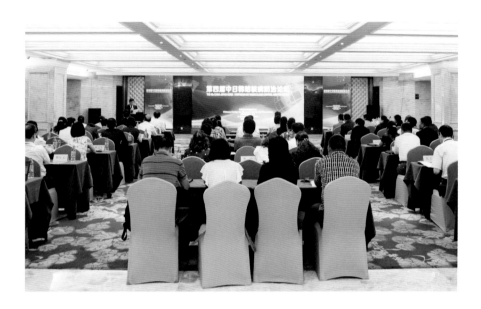

中、日、韩合作交流
Exchanges and cooperation among China, Japan, and South Korea

为建立中、日、韩三国间结核病疫情信息通报网络、协同开展跨境传染病防控工作，由中国疾病预防控制中心牵头，联合日本防痨协会结核病研究所、韩国结核病防治研究所，自2015年9月起建立每年轮换开展学术研讨的工作机制，以学术交流促进三国结防工作的发展。

To establish a trilateral network of tuberculosis monitoring among China, Japan, and South Korea and jointly carry out cross-border prevention and control of infectious diseases, a working mechanism to rotate an annual academic symposium in the three countries was formalized in September 2015, led by the Chinese Center for Disease Control and Prevention in partnership with the Japanese Research Institute of Tuberculosis and the Korean Institute of Tuberculosis. The program seeks to promote further progress on TB prevention and control in the three countries through academic exchanges.

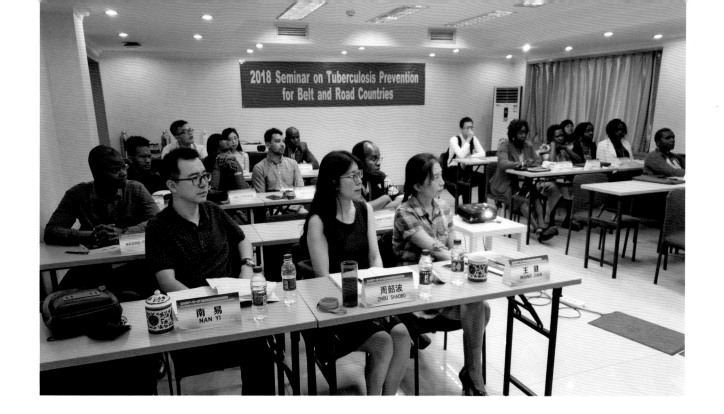

"一带一路"沿线国家合作交流

Cooperation and exchanges among Belt and Road countries

与此同时，中国也积极与"一带一路"沿线国家开展结核病防控工作的研讨、交流。举办"中国－中亚结核病控制论坛"，建立"中国－中亚结核病控制研修基地"，与巴基斯坦、马来西亚等国签署结核病防控战略合作协议。

At the same time, China is also actively conducting discussions and exchanges on tuberculosis prevention and control with countries in the Belt and Road Initiative (BRI). The China-Central Asia Tuberculosis Control Forum was held; the China-Central Asia Tuberculosis Control Training Facility was built; strategic cooperation agreements on the prevention and control of tuberculosis were signed with countries such as Pakistan and Malaysia.

2013—2019年，在商务部和国家卫生健康委国际交流与合作中心的支持下，成功举办12期结核病防治援外培训班和相关的高级研修班，先后培训了来自肯尼亚、毛里求斯、厄立特里亚、埃塞俄比亚、马拉维、赞比亚、苏丹、乌干达、桑给巴尔、塞拉利昂、博茨瓦纳、津巴布韦、朝鲜、冈比亚、南苏丹、印度尼西亚、洪都拉斯、摩尔多瓦、瓦努阿图、莱索托、阿塞拜疆、墨西哥、蒙古国、伊拉克、南非、埃及、利比里亚、巴基斯坦、巴勒斯坦、东帝汶、菲律宾、吉尔吉斯斯坦、柬埔寨、老挝、马尔代夫、马来西亚、孟加拉国、缅甸、斯里兰卡、泰国、文莱、也门、越南等43个国家的200多名结核病领域的防治官员和医务人员。

From 2013 to 2019, with the support of Chinese Ministry of Commerce (MOFCOM) and International exchange and cooperation center of National Health Commission (NHC), a total of twelve training courses and seminars were successfully organized. The trainees, over 200 TB control officials and medical staff in total, came from 43 Asian and African countries including Kenya, Mauritius, Eritrea, Ethiopia, Malawi, Zambia, Sultan, Uganda, Zanzibar, Sierra Leone, Botswana, Zimbabwe, North Korea, Gambia, South Sudan, Gambia, Indonesia, China, Iraq, South Africa, Egypt, Liberia, Pakistan, Palestine, East Timor, Philippines, Kyrgyzstan, Cambodia, Laos, Maldives, Malaysia, Bangladesh, Myanmar, Sri Lanka, Thailand, Brunei, Yemen, Vietnam.

古谚语云"他山之石，可以攻玉"，借助对外交流和对外培训，中国和亚洲、非洲多国可以互相砥砺、彼此学习，在结核病防控工作上协同发展！

Ancient Chinese wisdom states "stones from another mountain can polish jade". Through international exchanges and training programs, China, Asia, and Africa can learn from each other, reinforce efforts mutually, and coordinate their efforts on the prevention and control of tuberculosis!

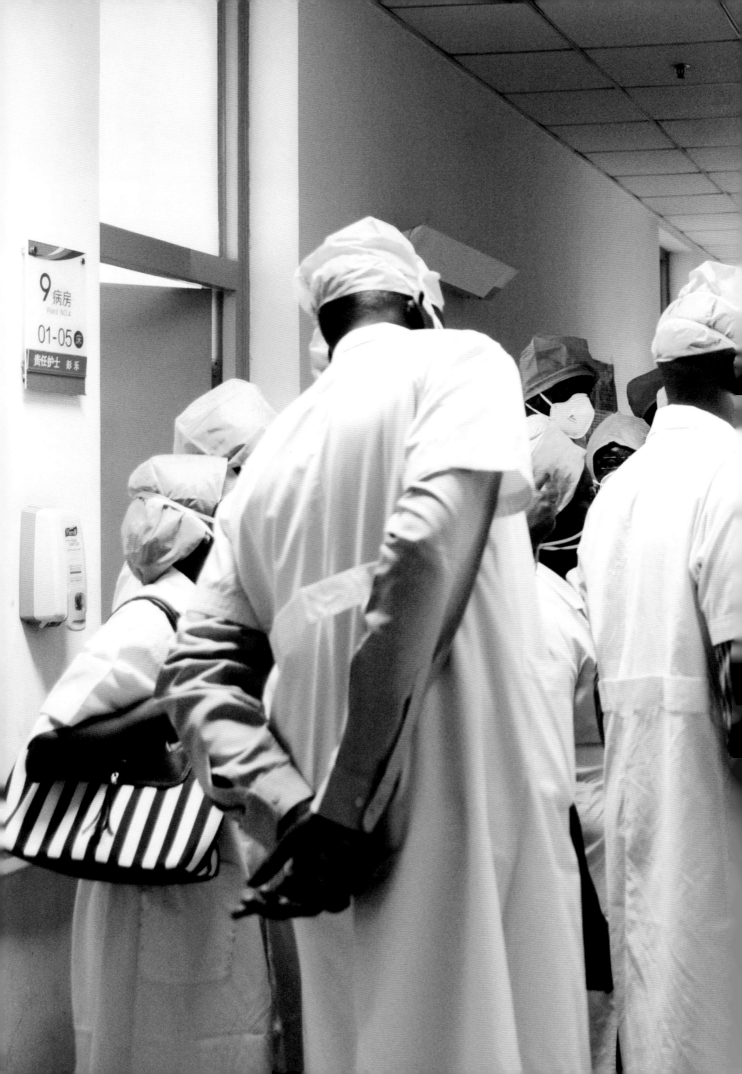

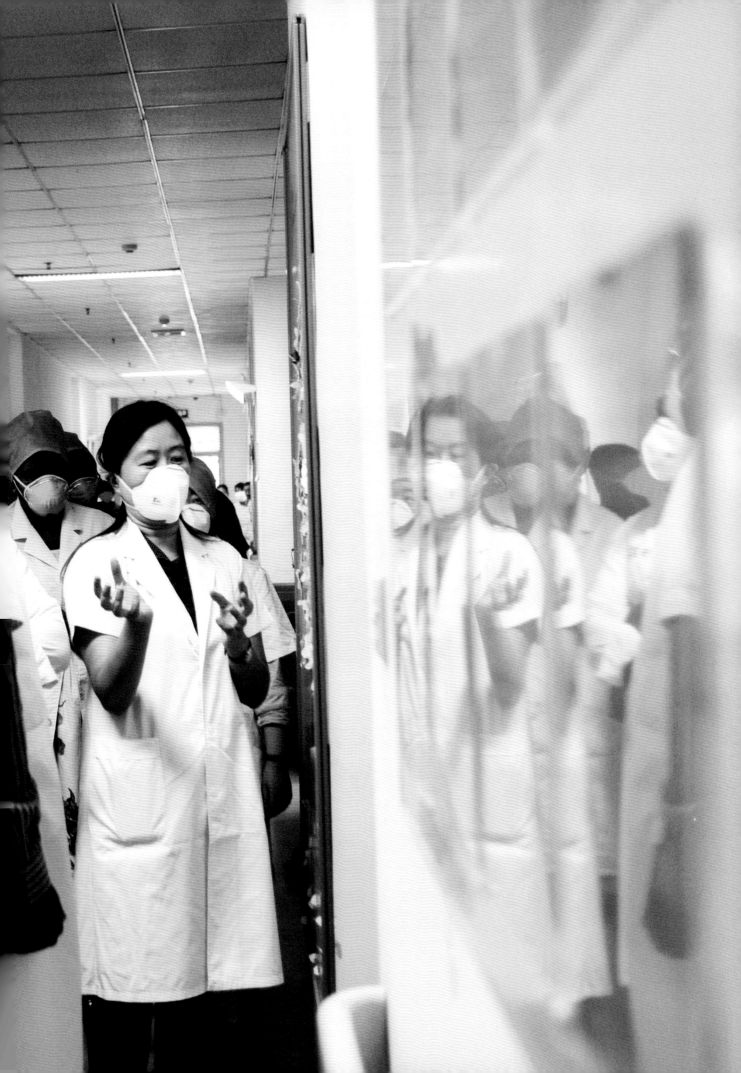

第七章

健康促进
全民参与

Chapter 7

Health Promotion
and Universal
Participation

中国结核病防治健康促进策略是"政府倡导、社会动员、健康教育",本着对公众普及结核病防治知识、提高结核病患者治疗依从、落实重点人群防控、营造良好社会氛围、提升政府关注支持的出发点,中国多年来持续开展丰富多彩的结核病防治健康促进和教育活动,通过多渠道、多主题、多手段动员全社会力量参与,在提高公众结核病防治知识知晓率、提升患者发现率等方面取得了显著成效。

China's health promotion strategy for tuberculosis prevention and control is "government advocacy, social mobilization, and health education". With the aim of popularizing the knowledge of tuberculosis prevention and control, increasing treatment adherence among tuberculosis patients, implementing prevention and control strategies among high-risk populations, creating a positive social atmosphere, and raising the attention and support of the government, China has carried out a variety of activities over the years. Through multiple channels, themes, and methods, China has mobilized participation from all the stakeholders and achieved remarkable results in improving the case finding rate and raising public awareness of tuberculosis prevention and control.

集中宣传与日常宣传相结合
Combining routine communication with campaigns

每年以 3 月 24 日"世界防治结核病日"为契机,在全国持续开展各类主题宣传活动,与媒体联合,面向大众宣传结核病防治核心信息,以点带面,覆盖各类人群,并把此项活动贯穿全年。

Every year on March 24th, World Tuberculosis Day is used as an opportunity to carry out nationwide thematic campaigns, with the media, to disseminate key messages around tuberculosis prevention and control to the general public. The goal is to engage all segments of the population and raise awareness throughout the year.

传统方式与新媒体相结合
Combining traditional approaches with new media

在广泛以传统方式,如海报、标语、墙报、广播、电视等宣传方式的基础上,与时俱进,紧紧与新媒体结合,开设微信、微博等官方账号,面向公众和专业人员开展宣传。官方微信公众号"结核那些事儿"成为全国疾控系统具有较大影响力的单病传播平台。

To keep pace with the times, new forms of communication are being employed based on the traditional publicity routes such as posters, slogans, wall posters, radio, television, etc. Such deployment is coordinated in alignment with new media. Publicity efforts are made through official accounts on platforms such as WeChat and Weibo to influence both professionals and the public. The official WeChat account "All about tuberculosis" became a significant communication platform within the national Disease Prevention and Control system for a single disease.

专业宣传与志愿者宣传相结合
Combining informational campaigns and volunteer advocacy

在充分借助各级各类专业人员宣传的基础上，充分开展全国"百千万志愿者结核病防治知识传播活动"，鼓励社会各界人士自愿参与到结核病防治宣传队伍中，主动开展结核病防治知识的宣传。目前，公益志愿者队伍已多达90余万人。

To make full use of publicity at all sectors and levels, China has waged a campaign for millions of volunteers to spread knowledge about tuberculosis prevention and control throughout the country. People from all walks of life are encouraged to volunteer on the TB prevention and control publicity team and to proactively disseminate TB prevention and control knowledge. At present, there are more than 900,000 volunteers.

开发和更新健康教育资源库
Enriching and updating the health education resource bank

针对不同人群文化特点，开发和更新内容丰富、形式多样的传播资料，建立了中国结核病防治健康教育资源库，涵盖了文字、图片、音频、视频等各种形式的结核病防治知识传播材料，资源库还获得国际防痨与肺部疾病联盟颁发的奖项。多年来全国各地也涌现出众多的优秀科普作品，惠及了当地的结核病健康宣传工作。资源库在实现对公众宣传的全面覆盖以及对重点人群的精准宣传等方面发挥了重要的作用。宣传资料还被编译多种语言，在民族地区广泛使用。

A diverse set of communication materials targeting different groups were developed in various formats based on sub-culture characteristics. A resource bank was developed for TB prevention and control in China, which includes texts, images, audio, video, and other forms of TB informational materials. The resource bank has also won an award from the International Union Against Tuberculosis and Lung Disease. Over the years, many outstanding TB science popularization works have been developed across the country, benefiting local TB control efforts. The resource bank is vital to achieving universal publicity coverage and targeted communication with key populations. The informational materials were also synthesized and translated for use in ethnic areas.

3·24世界防治结核病日，中国在行动

CHINA IN ACTION: MARCH 24TH, THE WORLD TUBERCULOSIS DAY

每年的3月24日是世界防治结核病日（World Tuberculosis Day），旨在提高全球对结核病负担以及预防工作的认识，提升政治和社会承诺，向终止结核病进一步努力。

Every year on March 24th, World Tuberculosis Day, efforts are made to raise global awareness of the burden of tuberculosis, to promote prevention efforts, and to elevate political and public commitments for making further efforts to end TB.

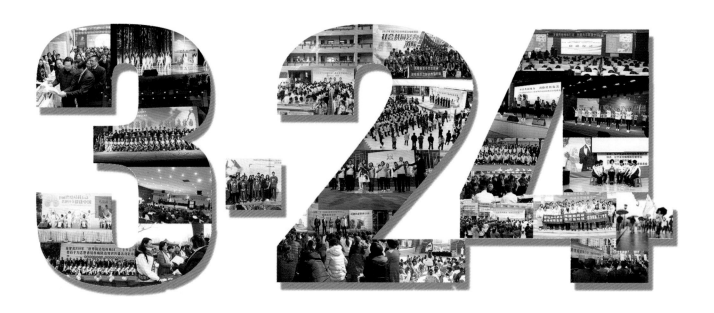

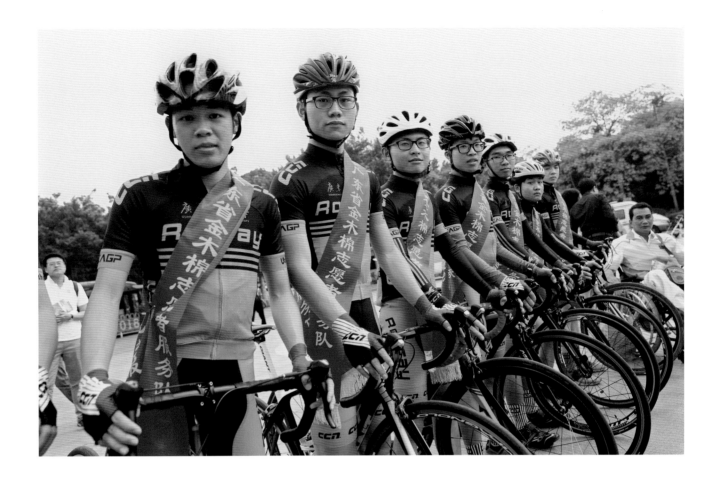

这个特殊纪念日的来源要追溯到130多年前。1882年3月24日，德国微生物学家罗伯特·科赫宣布结核分枝杆菌是导致结核病的病原菌，1995年底，世界卫生组织为了进一步唤起公众与结核病作斗争的意识，将每年的3月24日确立为世界防治结核病日（World Tuberculosis Day）。

The origin of this special commemorative day dates back more than 130 years. On March 24th, 1882, German microbiologist Robert Koch declared mycobacterium is the pathogen causing tuberculosis. At the end of 1995, the World Health Organization (WHO) formalized March 24th each year as World Tuberculosis Day to further raise public awareness of the fight against TB.

每年的3·24世界防治结核病日期间，全国各级卫生健康部门都要组织开展丰富多彩的主题宣传日、宣传周和宣传月等系列大型倡导活动，向广大的公众传播结核病防治知识、倡导社会各界力量积极行动起来，采取有效措施，控制结核病疫情，消除结核病的社会危害，为实现健康中国共同努力。以此纪念日为引领，各级结核病防治有关的宣传活动贯穿全年。

Every year, during World Tuberculosis Day on March 24th, health departments at all levels throughout the country organize a wide range of advocacy activities and events, such as thematic awareness days, weeks, and months to spread knowledge about tuberculosis prevention and control to the general public. The activities may also include advocacy for all sectors of society to mobilize resources to take effective measures against tuberculosis epidemic, mitigate the social harm of the disease, and achieve the Healthy China goals. The events on World Tuberculosis Day will then set off a year-long effort of publicity and outreach on tuberculosis prevention and control.

多种宣传工具，助力健康促进

MULTIPLE PUBLICITY TOOLS TO PROMOTE HEALTH AWARENESS

工欲善其事、必先利其器。多年来，广大的各级结核病防治工作者充分利用专业知识和才艺智慧，设计、开发和制作了众多通俗易懂和公众喜闻乐见的科普作品与宣传工具，发放到不同受众手中，成为他们自身开展学习和对外宣传倡导的重要载体。

To increase work productivity, one must first sharpen the tools. Over the years, the vast number of tuberculosis health professionals at all levels have made full use of their knowledge, skills, and creativity to design, develop, and produce a wide range of popular science works and publicity tools. These tools are easy to understand and popular with the public, allowing for distribution across different audiences. Such tools have become an important vehicle for independent learning, public advocacy, and outreach.

健康教育资源库

Health education resource bank

历年来，国家和地方各级设计开发了多种多样的科普宣传作品，供各地开展结核病防治宣传教育活动使用。此外还制作了针对不同人群的多种传播材料，如农村居民、学生、流动人口、医务人员、肺结核患者和家属、结核菌/艾滋病病毒双重感染者等，这些宣传材料在全国结核病防治健康教育工作中发挥了巨大的作用。

Over the years, a wide variety of science popularization works have been designed and developed at the national and local levels for tuberculosis education campaigns. Additionally, targeted communication materials have been produced for different groups, such as rural residents, students, migrant populations, medical personnel, families of tuberculosis patients, and people with HIV/TB co-infection. These materials have played an important role in health education for the prevention and control of tuberculosis throughout the country.

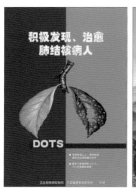 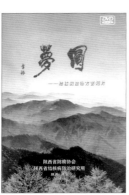 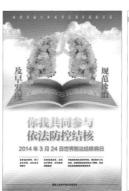 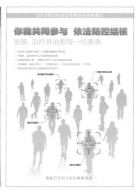 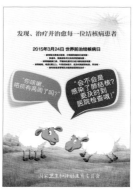

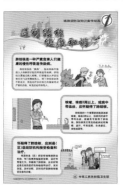 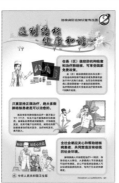 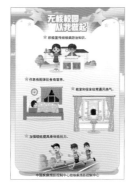 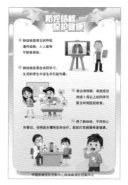 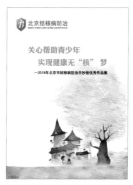

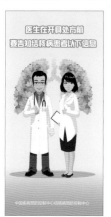 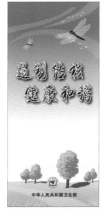 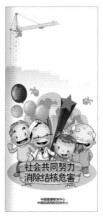 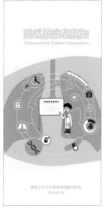 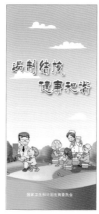 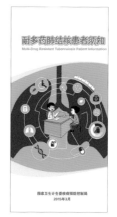

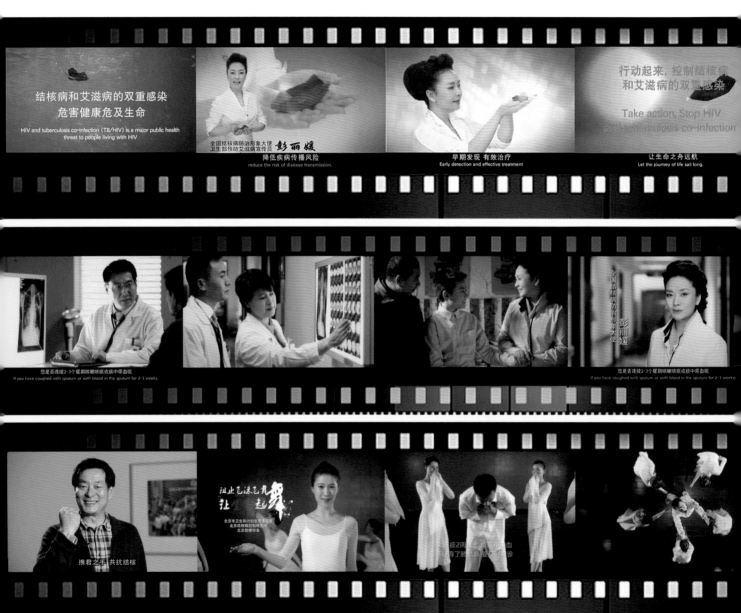

结核病防治公益广告
Public service advertisement on TB control

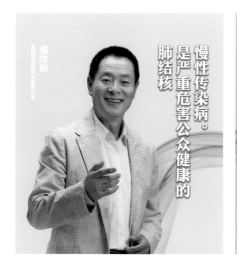

慢性传染病。
是严重危害公众健康的
肺结核

潘存昕
全国城市结核病宣传大使

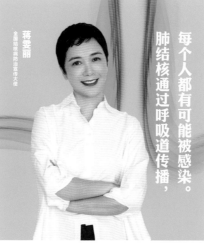

每个人都有可能被感染。
肺结核通过呼吸道传播，

蒋雯丽
全国结核病防治宣传大使

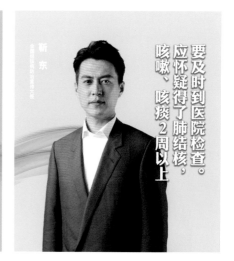

要及时到医院检查。
应怀疑得了肺结核，
咳嗽、咳痰2周以上

靳东
全国结核病防治宣传大使

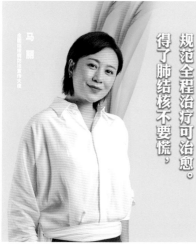

规范全程治疗可治愈。
得了肺结核不要慌，

马丽
全国结核病防治宣传大使

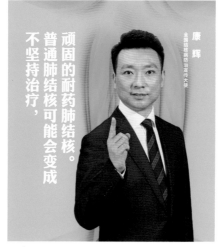

顽固的耐药肺结核。
普通肺结核可能会变成
不坚持治疗，

康辉
全国结核病防治宣传大使

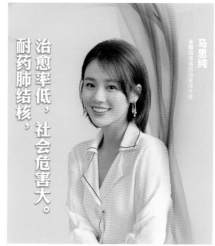

治愈率低，社会危害大。
耐药肺结核，

马思纯
全国结核病防治宣传大使

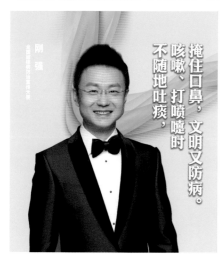

掩住口鼻，文明又防病。
咳嗽、打喷嚏时
不随地吐痰，

刚强
全国结核病防治宣传大使

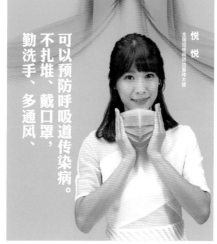

可以预防呼吸道传染病。
不扎堆、戴口罩、
勤洗手、多通风、

悦悦
全国结核病防治宣传大使

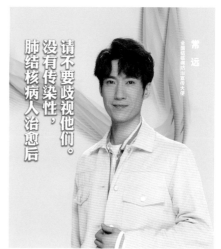

请不要歧视他们。
没有传染性，
肺结核病人治愈后

常远
全国慢性病防治宣传大使

结核病防治海报
TB control posters

面对面宣传教育
Face-to-face communication and education

张大爷今天出门办事回来，小区外面围了一群人，原来是市疾控中心的医务人员在做结核病宣传。张大爷凑过去拿了一张宣传单想了解一下，医务人员赶紧走过来跟他攀谈起来。医生问他是否知道肺结核，家里有人得过肺结核吗？知道肺结核是通过什么方式传染的吗……说着说着就打开了话匣子，张大爷逐一回答了问题，还提出了不少问题，比如平时要注意什么呀？有症状了要去哪里检查等，一场谈话下来，张大爷觉得自己对结核病的知识比以前知道得更多了，还澄清了许多错误认识。面对面的结核病防治知识宣传，可以起到事半功倍的作用！

Uncle ZHANG, on his way home, saw a group of people gathered around the health workers of the municipal CDC, who were having publicity of tuberculosis knowledge. ZHANG walked to the group and picked up a leaflet. One health worker hurried over to talk to him. The doctor asked if he knew about tuberculosis. Did anyone in his family have tuberculosis? Didhe know TB's transmission route? While talking, ZHANG answered the questions one-by-one and also raised many questions. For example, what should he do to prevent tuberculosis? If he developed symptoms, where should he go for a check-up? ZHANG felt he learned more about tuberculosis than before and cleared up many misunderstandings after the conversation. Face-to-face communication about tuberculosis prevention and control can really maximize the impact of education.

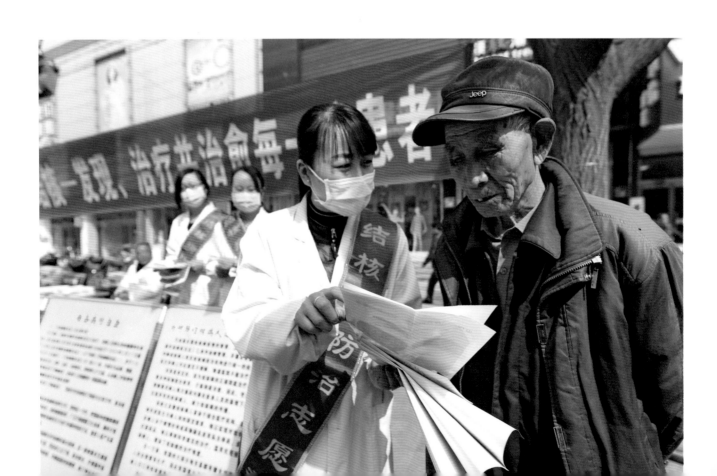

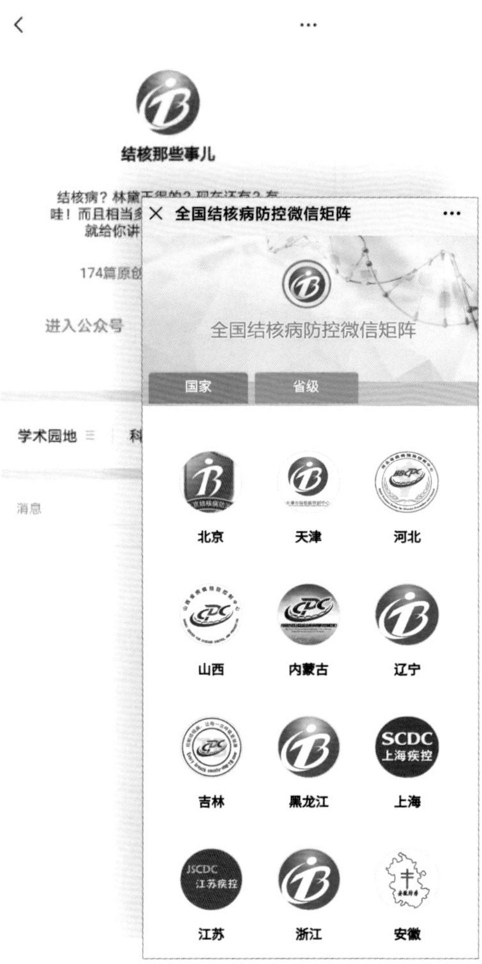

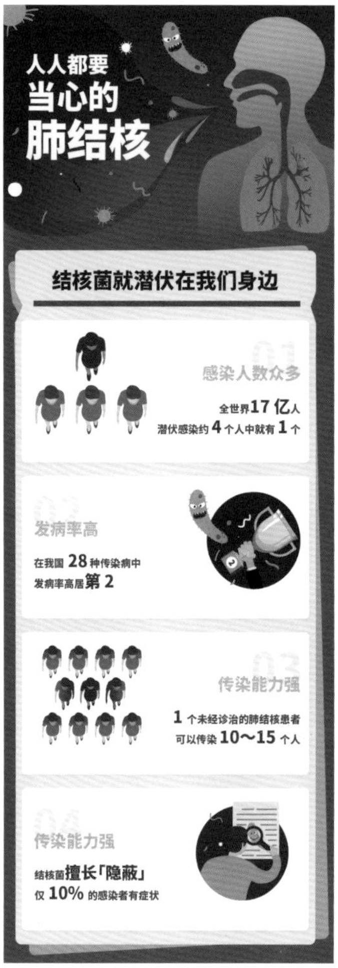

请扫描二维码，了解更多结核病防治知识
Please scan the QR code to learn more about tuberculosis control.

结核病官方微信号
WeChat account for TB control

新媒体探索
New media experiments

国家层面建立了“一网一微”的主流宣传平台，即“中国结核网”和“结核那些事儿”微信公众号，成为学习业务知识、普及防治科普、掌握政策动向的重要载体，惠及了全国数以万计的结核病防治工作者和广大百姓。2018年，创建了与全国31个省（自治区、直辖市）互联互通的结核病防治微信矩阵平台，开创单病公众号联动宣传先河，极大地拓展了全国结核病防治新媒体的宣传效应。

At the national level, a “China Tuberculosis” website and the “All about Tuberculosis” WeChat account constitute the mainstream publicity platforms. They serve as important access points for gaining technical knowledge as well as outlets for popularizing TB science and sources for tracking policy updates. The platforms have benefited tens of thousands of tuberculosis workers and the general public throughout the country. In 2018, the Tuberculosis Control and Prevention WeChat matrix platform was established with interconnectivity among all 31 Chinese provinces (municipalities and autonomous regions). It set a precedent for coordinated publicity efforts on WeChat around a single disease and greatly extended the publicity impact of tuberculosis prevention and control in new media.

结核病防治"从娃娃抓起"

Tuberculosis awareness building with

children

11岁的亮亮（化名）读小学五年级，放学后妈
妈觉得他与往日有些不同。比如一回家就赶紧
去洗手、漱口；吃饭时爷爷打了一个喷嚏，他
还义正言辞地告诉爷爷打喷嚏时要背过身去捂
住口鼻；爸爸咳嗽了几声他又赶快过来嘘寒问
暖。妈妈忍不住问亮亮，这到底是怎么回事？

Liang Liang, an 11-year-old boy, is in fifth grade
in primary school. His mom found something
different about her son after school. Liang Liang
went straight to the bathroom to wash his hands
and rinse his mouth. At dinner, grandpa sneezed
and Liang Liang immediately told him to turn his
head and cover his nose and mouth. When dad
coughed a few times, Liang Liang quickly came
up to check on him. His behavior was really
different. Mom could not help asking him what
was happening.

原来，亮亮今天在学校上了一堂健康教育课，
内容是介绍结核病预防知识的。他听得认真，
回家后还活学活用。2016年，结核病防治知识
正式纳入到了黑龙江省九年义务教育地方课程
《生命教育》五年级（下）课本中，此举备受
师生和家长的认可与赞同。

It turned out that Liang Liang attended a health
education class at school, where he was
introduced to the information on tuberculosis
prevention. He listened carefully and came
home to apply what he had learned. In 2016, the
tuberculosis prevention and control information
was officially incorporated into the textbook "Life
Education" for the fifth grade (second semester)
students in Heilongjiang province as part of the
nine-year compulsory education. This move was
applauded by teachers, students, and parents.

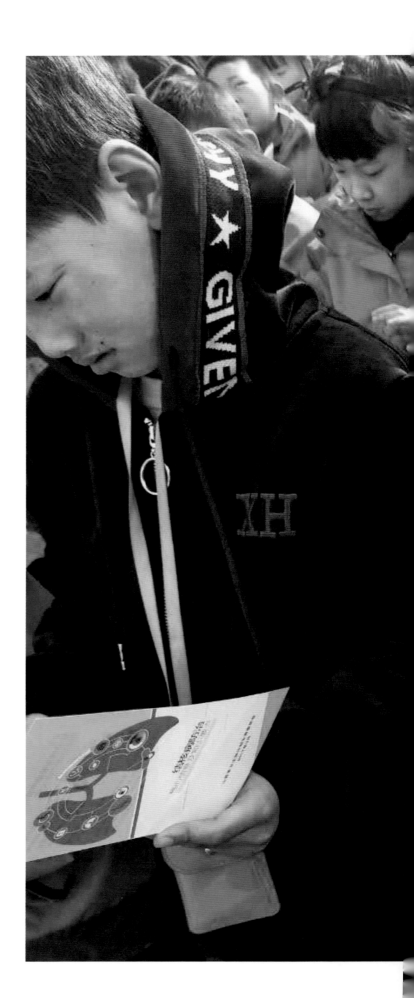

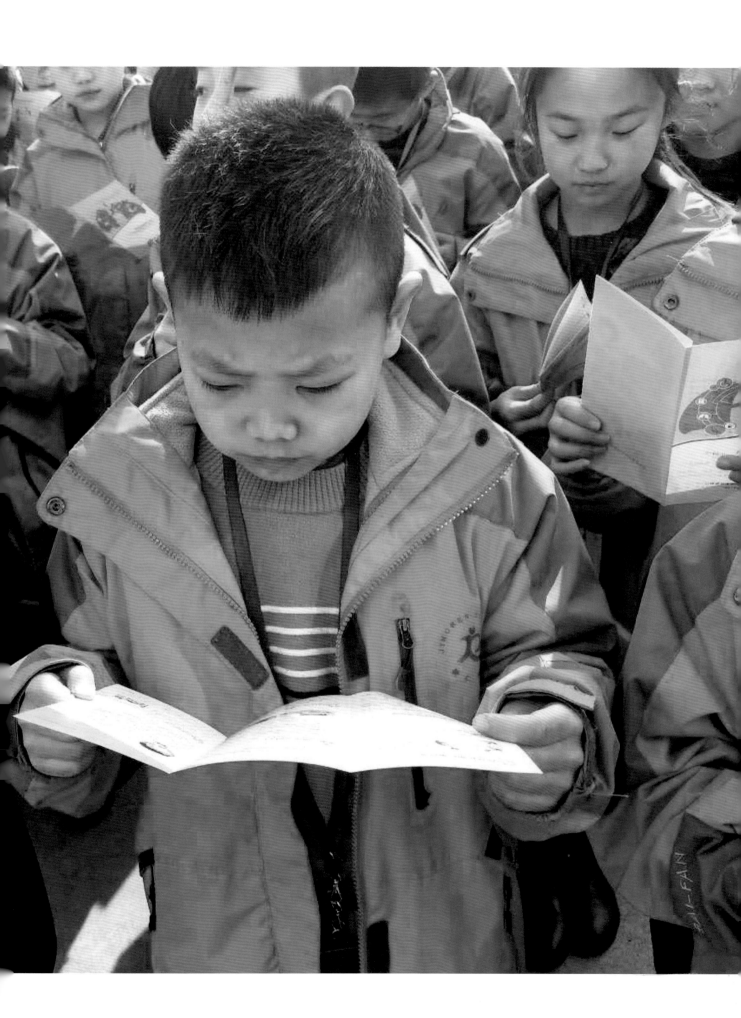

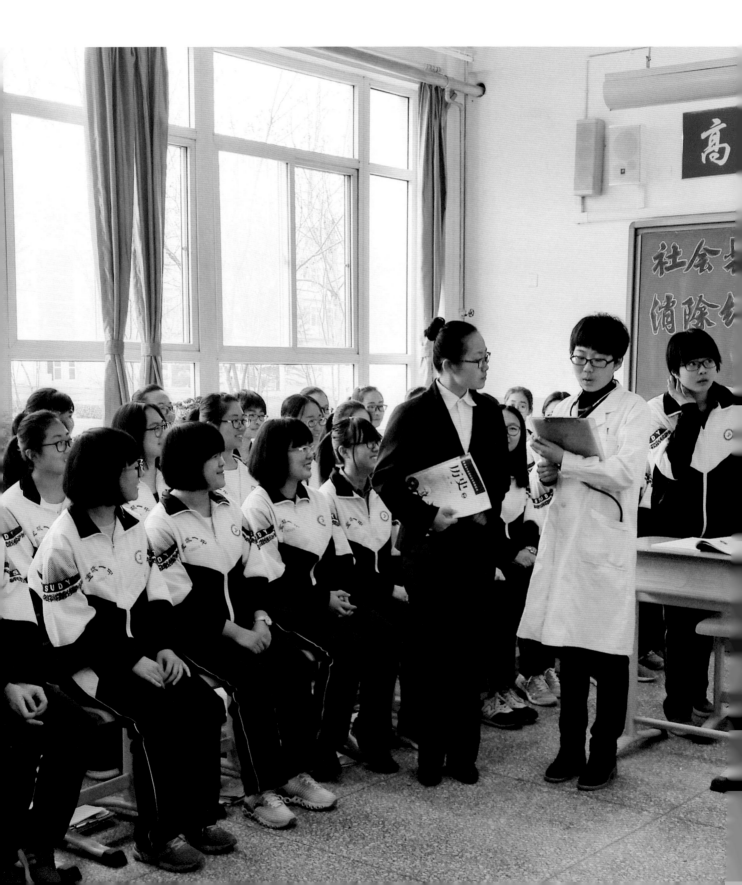

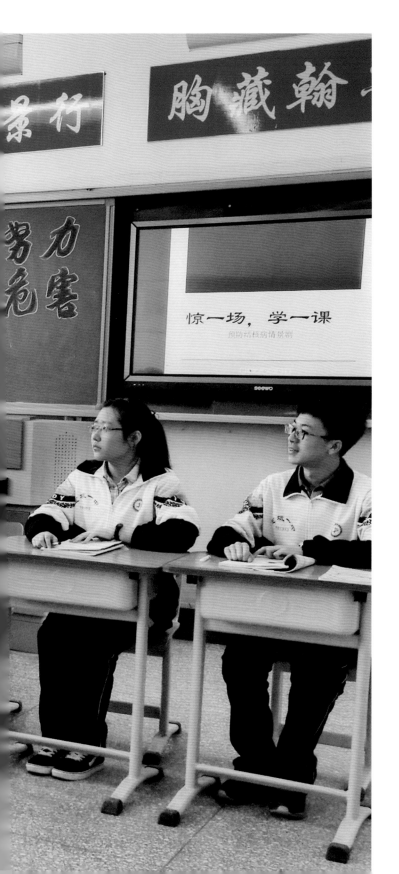

宣传形式异彩纷呈
A variety of knowledge aware building events

知识普及：知识竞赛、网络游戏、宣讲比赛、谜语竞猜、科普演讲、技术练兵等。
Knowledge popularization: knowledge games, online games, speaking competitions, quizzes and riddles, popular science lectures, and technical training, etc.

表演创作：话剧、情景剧、方言剧、地方戏曲、文艺汇演等。
Creative performance: dramas, role plays, dialect dramas, local operas, variety shows, etc.

文艺创作：手工绘本、漫画大赛等。
Literary and artistic creation: hand-painted books and cartoon contests, etc.

户外宣传：徒步行、摩托车比赛、迷你马拉松、共享单车等。
Outdoor activities: hikes, motorcycle races, mini-marathons, bike sharing, etc.

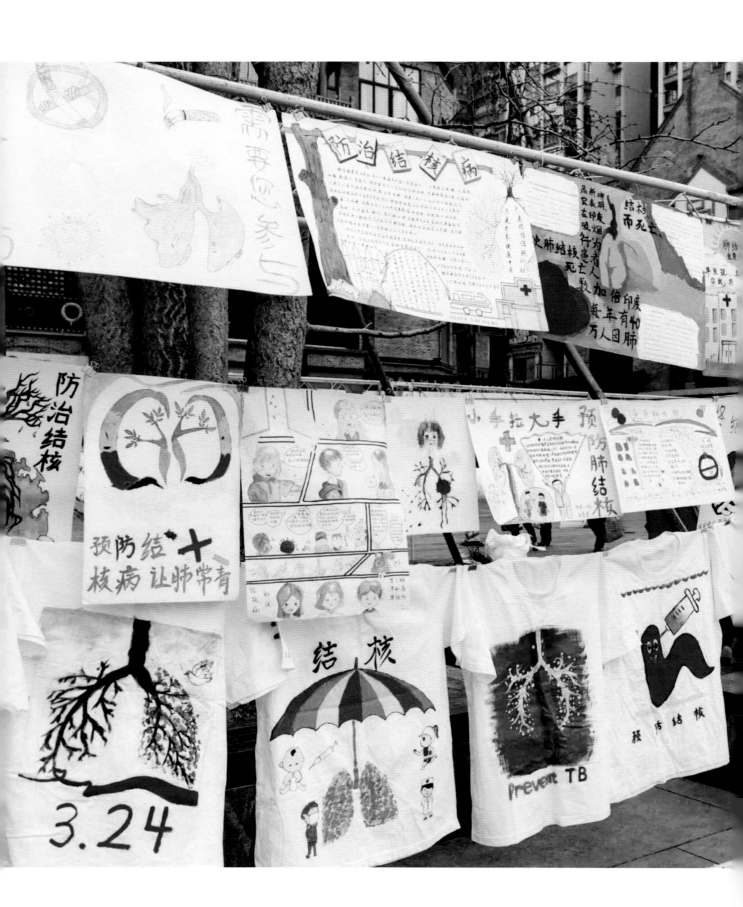

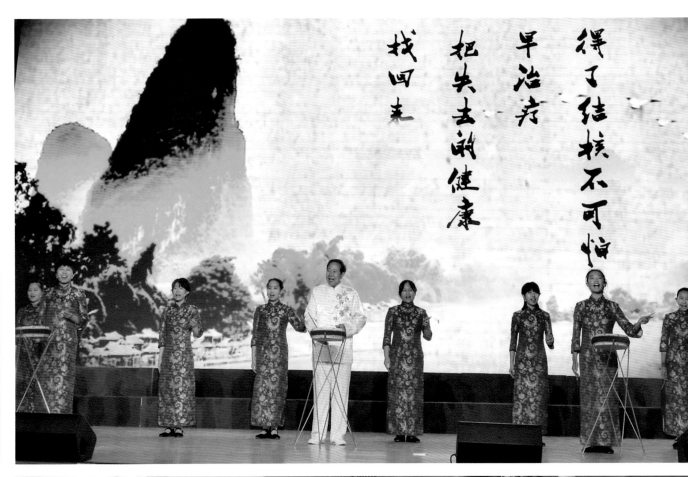

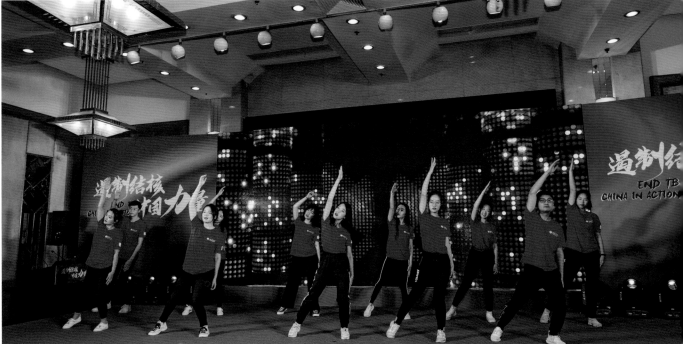

百千万志愿者的公益力量

THE PUBLIC SERVICE POWER OF MILLIONS OF VOLUNTEERS

为广泛发动社会力量开展结核病防治知识普及宣传，2012年3月，全国"百千万志愿者结核病防治知识传播行动"（简称"百千万行动"）拉开序幕，逐步形成全社会结核病防治知识的传播链，是中国结核病防治健康促进工作的一大特色。目前，全国已有90余万志愿者，他们像春风里播洒而出的蒲公英种子，在各地生根发芽，用自己的努力和付出给更多人带去知识、关爱和力量。

In order to mobilize social actors to spread the knowledge about tuberculosis prevention and control, a nationwide "Millions of Volunteers Tuberculosis Prevention Knowledge Dissemination" campaign (referred to as the Million Volunteers campaign) kicked off in March 2012, gradually forming a society-wide chain of tuberculosis prevention and control knowLedge dissemination network. Nowadays, there are more than 900,000 volunteers in the country. They are like dandelion seeds that spread in the spring breeze, which take root and sprout in all parts of the country, to bring knowledge, care, and strength to, more people with their efforts.

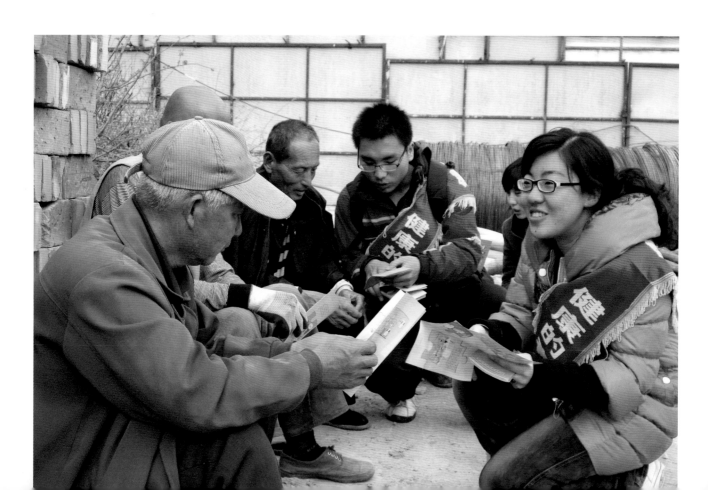

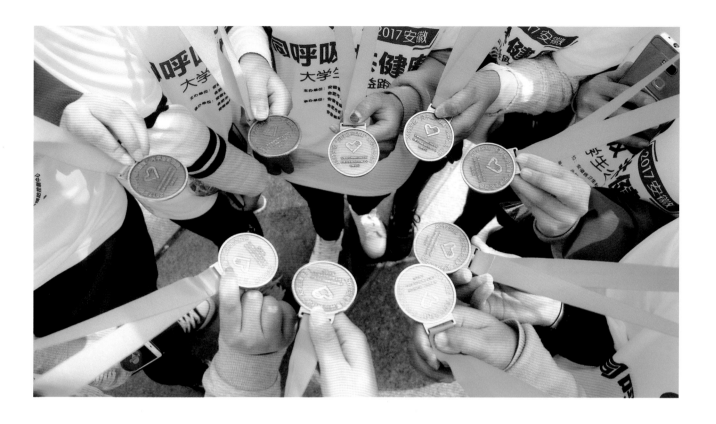

团体培育，基地建设

Volunteer training and training base construction

安徽省从2015起建立薪火相传大学生志愿者团体培育计划，以实施性项目形式招募和发展志愿者，目前已在全省组建了74支志愿者队伍，覆盖安徽省一半以上高校。天津市自2012年起创建大学生志愿者健康教育科普示范基地，组建结核病防治宣传队伍，常年活跃在全市各区，并带动各区建立了区级宣传教育基地，又进一步把活动经验辐射到社区，建立了社区宣教基地，形成市、区和基层社区的宣传网。

Beginning in 2015, Anhui Province established the Trail-blazer volunteering grooming program to help recruit and develop volunteers through project implementation. So far, 74 volunteer groups have been formed throughout the province, covering more than half of the universities in Anhui. In 2012, Tianjin Municipality set up a health education and science demonstration base to train college students as mobile volunteers of health education and outreach for tuberculosis control. These volunteers have been actively driving the establishment of district-level facilities for health education. They introduced new practices to the community level and helped create the community-level infrastructure. Now, a comprehensive publicity network extending from the municipal level down to the community level is fully functional.

徒步宣传，为健康行走

Hiking for health

山东省滕州市组建的"滕州徒步，为健康行走"志愿者组织，是中国第一个把徒步健身运动与百千万志愿者行动结合在一起的民间社团组织，目前已成立60多支宣传队伍，志愿者达1万多人。这些志愿者是各行各业的工作人员，他们连续性地开展把徒步健身、宣传结核病防治知识，贫困救助融为一体的公益活动，向公众传播健康、奉献和互助理念，形成城市的一道亮丽风景线。

The Hiking for Health volunteer group, organized by Tengzhou city, Shandong province, is the first civil society organization in China that combines hiking fitness exercise with millions of volunteer activities for tuberculosis control. So far, 60 advocacy teams have been formed with more than 10,000 volunteers.These volunteers come from all walks of life. They carried out a series of charitable activities with themes ranging from tuberculosis prevention and control knowledge to poverty relief. With the motto of health, dedication and mutual support.

昔日结核病患，如今宣传使者

Advocates and educators out of cured TB patients

患有肺结核的"嘟嘟"是结核病患者互助平台"百度肺结核吧"的吧主。这是一个结核病患者的互助之家，也是一个宣传结核病防治知识的网络公益平台。"百度肺结核吧"2011年建立，如今已有9万贴吧会员，发帖数量超过1 000万。除了线上为结核病病友答疑解惑，还积极在线下组织丰富多彩的公益活动，足迹遍布祖国名山大川，并引起国际组织的关注和赞赏。

Dudu is the owner of the Baidu tuberculosis virtual home, a mutual support group for tuberculosis patients and an online non-profit platform to promote the tuberculosis prevention and control knowledge. Since the launch of this virtual community in 2011, its membership has grown to 90,000 with more than 10 million posts. In addition to answering questions for tuberculosis patients online, this group has also produced a variety of charitable activities and tours across China, attracting the attention and accolade of international organizations.

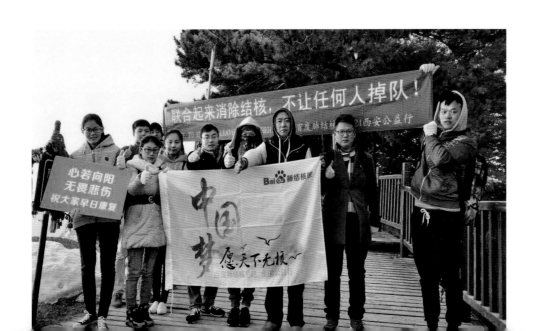

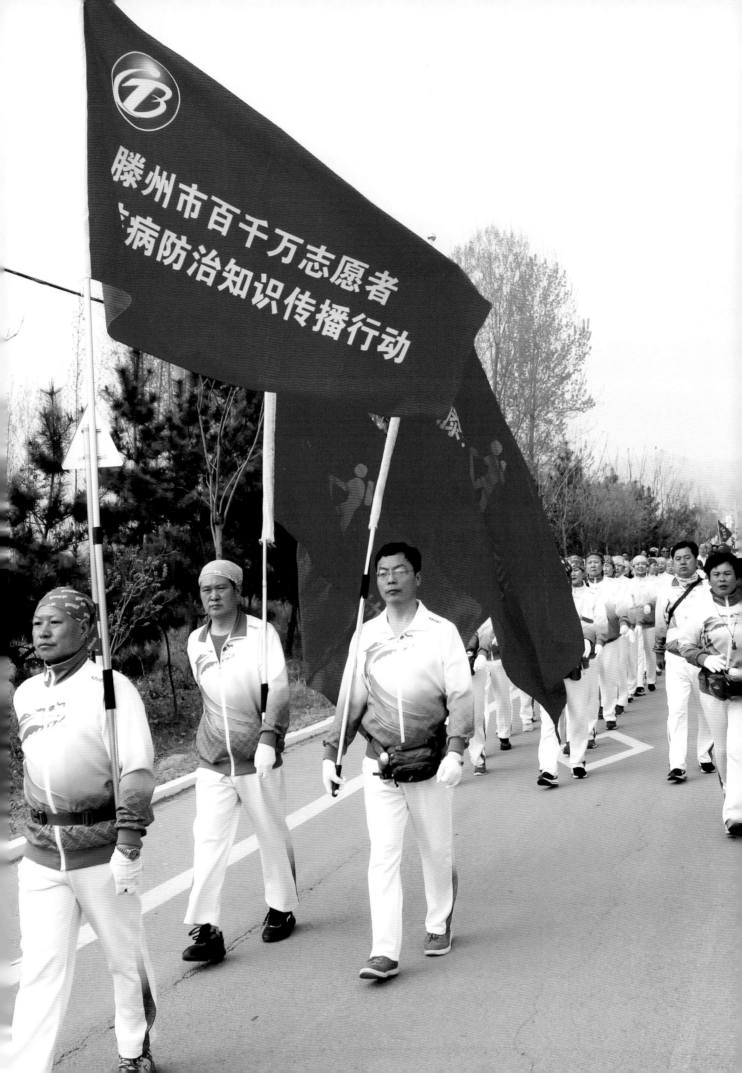

特区义工"赠人玫瑰，手有余香"

Volunteers in Shenzhen: belief in acts of kindness

有这样一群人，他们不计报酬，基于道义、信念、良知、同情心和责任，为改进社会服务，贡献着个人的时间、精力和技术特长，他们就是义工。深圳的义工志愿者在全国小有名气，他们身穿"红马甲"活跃于各个基层社区。如今义工志愿者的活动内容里又加入了结核病防治知识的宣传，他们不仅利用面对面、网络、微信、QQ群等形式进行宣传，还带动更多人加入志愿活动。政府还将义工结核病宣传活动时间计入义工工时，成为办理积分入户、子女积分入学的重要佐证材料。"赠人玫瑰，手有余香"，传递知识，共享健康，是义工志愿者们工作的日常写照。

There is a group of people who devote their time, energy, and expertise to improve public services without pay. Their acts of kindness, are based on morality, faith, conscience, compassion, and responsibility. They are volunteers in Shenzhen, wearing a red vest and active in every community, and have earned a reputation in China. Nowadays, the volunteers have developed activities of knowledge publicity awareness on tuberculosis prevention and control. The volunteers use face- to-face interactions, internet tools, and social media such as WeChat and QQ group to conduct outreach, while encouraging more people to volunteer. The government has also included the time spent on TB publicity activities into the working hours of volunteers, which can be used for resident permits and local school enrollment of volunteers' children. As it is said, a random act of kindness can make all the difference. Sharing knowledge and promoting universal health is the daily work of volunteers.

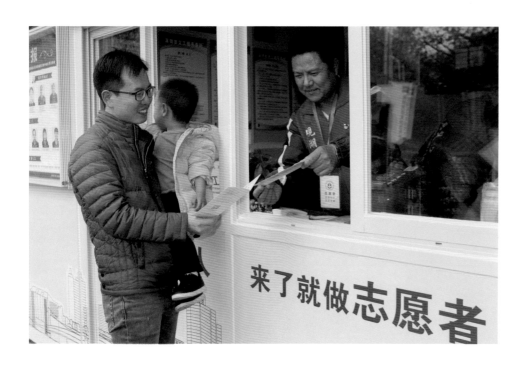

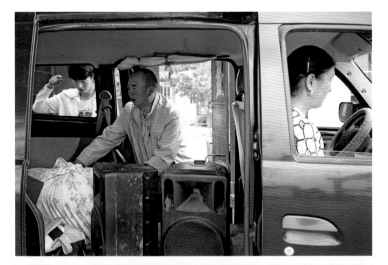

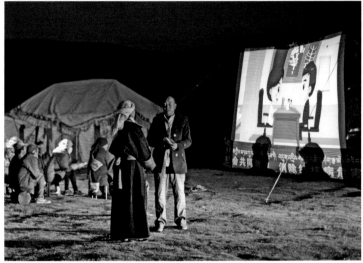

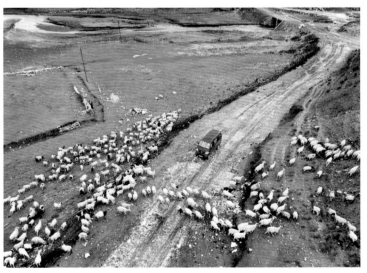

草原上的夫妻放映队
The film-screening couple on the prairie

在青海省海南藏族自治州共和县铁盖乡，住着一对家喻户晓的夫妻——许国强（化名）和马玉梅（化名）。他们是乡村电影放映员，更是结核病的宣传使者。

In Tiegai Village, Gongghe County, Qinghai Province, lives a well-known couple, XU Guoqiang and his wife MA Yumei. They tour the local villages to screen films where they also disseminate information on tuberculosis control.

许国强从1988年开始为农牧民们放映露天电影，每次放电影前都会放结核病防治宣传片，大概20多分钟，很受牧民、村民欢迎。他觉得这些东西有用，可惜自己懂得不多，便主动找到疾控中心要到更多的宣传资料。

XU began screening open-air movies for farmers and herdsmen in 1988. Before each screening, the couple would hold a tuberculosis prevention and control information session for about 20 minutes. Their screenings were very popular among the herders and villagers. XU felt that the tuberculosis information he was giving was useful, but he knew too little, so he went to the local CDC for more materials.

这些年做下来，许国强夫妇对结核病防治知识有了更深入的了解，对宣传的重要性也有了更深的体会。如今在当地疾控中心的支持下，他们的宣传材料更加丰富了，而且材料还被译成了少数民族文字，很受农牧民喜欢。

After many years, XU and MA have deepened their knowledge of tuberculosis prevention and control and their appreciation of the importance of publicity. With the support of the local CDC, their promotional materials have been plentiful and translated into ethnic languages. The programs remain very popular with farmers and herders.

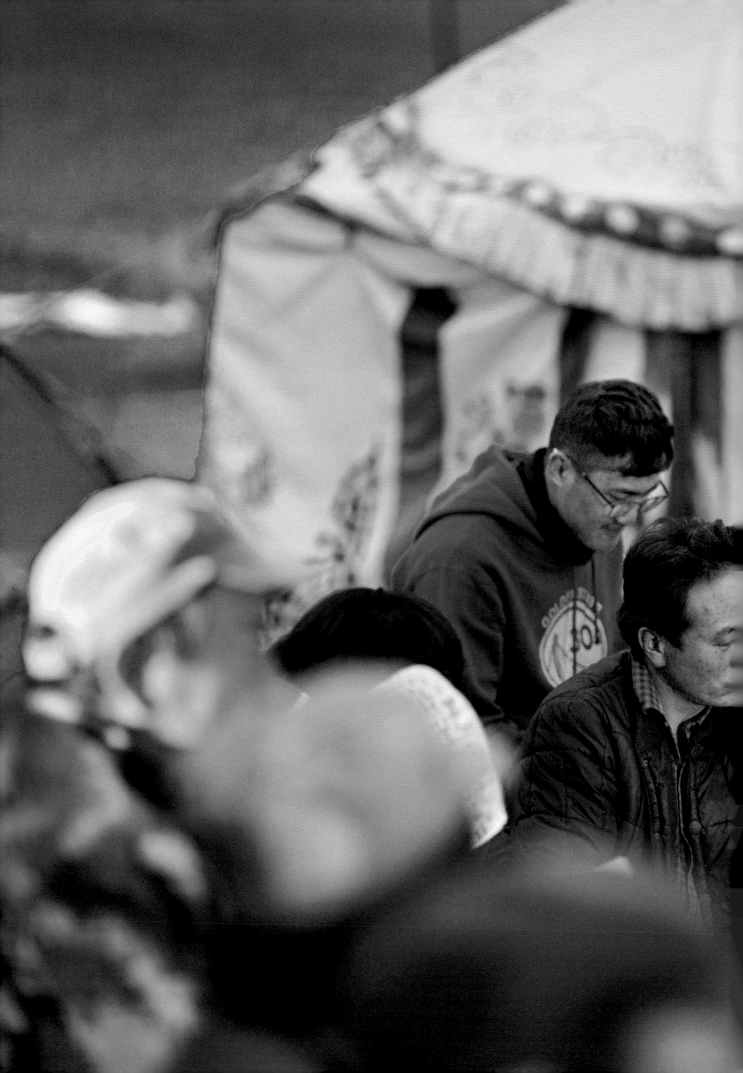

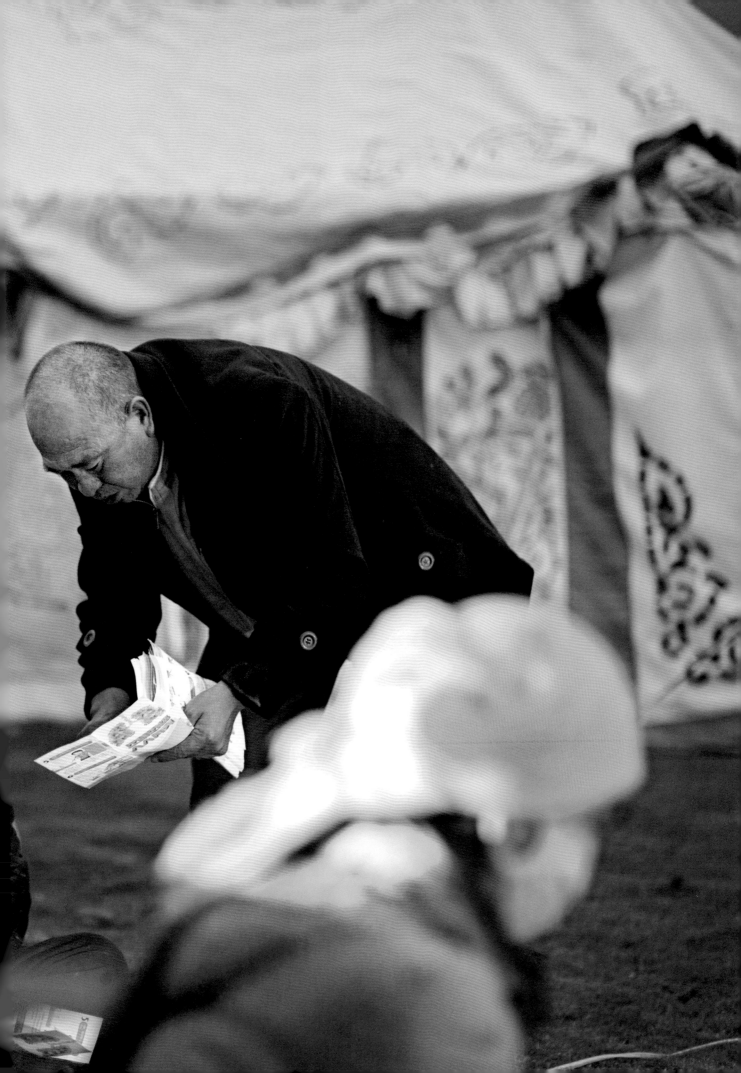

为终止结核病，点亮中国红

LIGHTING UP TO SHOW OUR DETERMINATION TO END TB

2018年9月26日，联合国大会在美国纽约联合国总部召开，同一天，联合国大会终止结核病问题高级别会议拉开序幕，这是全球抗击结核病历史上的里程碑事件，奏响为实现2030年全球终止结核病目标的新乐章！本次终止结核病高级别会议的主题是"团结一致终止结核病：全世界紧急应对这一全球性流行病"。向全球宣布加速行动终止结核病流行！

On September 26th, 2018, as the United Nations General Assembly was being held at the United Nations Headquarters in New York, USA, the United Nations high-level meeting on tuberculosis kicked off. This meeting was a milestone in the history of the global fight against TB and a new chapter in achieving the goal of ending tuberculosis globally by 2030. The theme of this high-level meeting was "united to end tuberculosis: an urgent global response to a global epidemic".

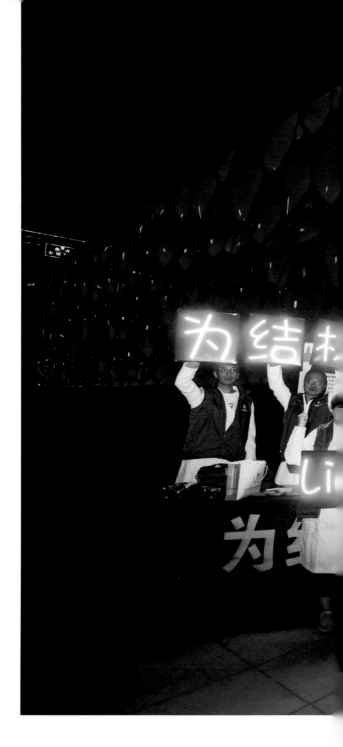

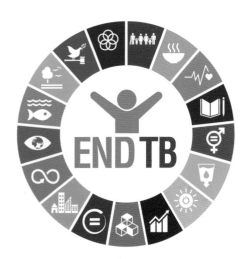

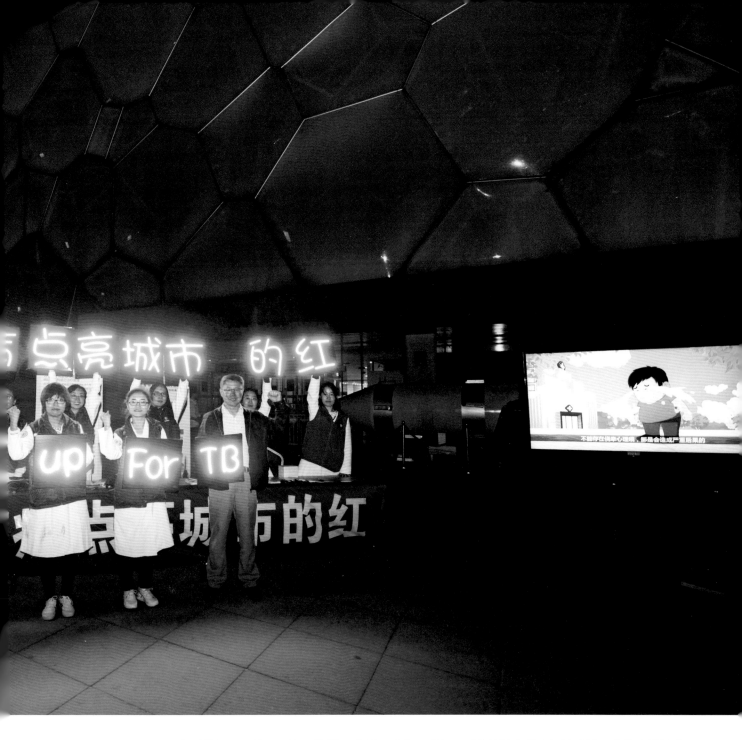

中国北京、天津、上海、杭州、广州、重庆、武汉、西安等城市的地标性建筑，为终止结核病的承诺而点亮成红！

Landmark buildings in the eight Chinese cities of Beijing, Tianjin, Shanghai, Hangzhou, Guangzhou, Chongqing, Wuhan and Xi'an lit up in red for the shared commitment to end tuberculosis!

北京
Beijing

国家游泳中心"水立方"（Water Cube），全球奥运健儿万马驰骋的辽阔疆场，它的周身被点亮成一抹浓浓的中国红，同时点亮了为抗击结核病而彰显的美好愿望和坚定决心！

The National Aquatics Center (Water Cube), a celebrated venue for global athletics during the 2008 Olympics, had its four facades illuminated in Chinese red to underscore the ambition and determination to end tuberculosis!

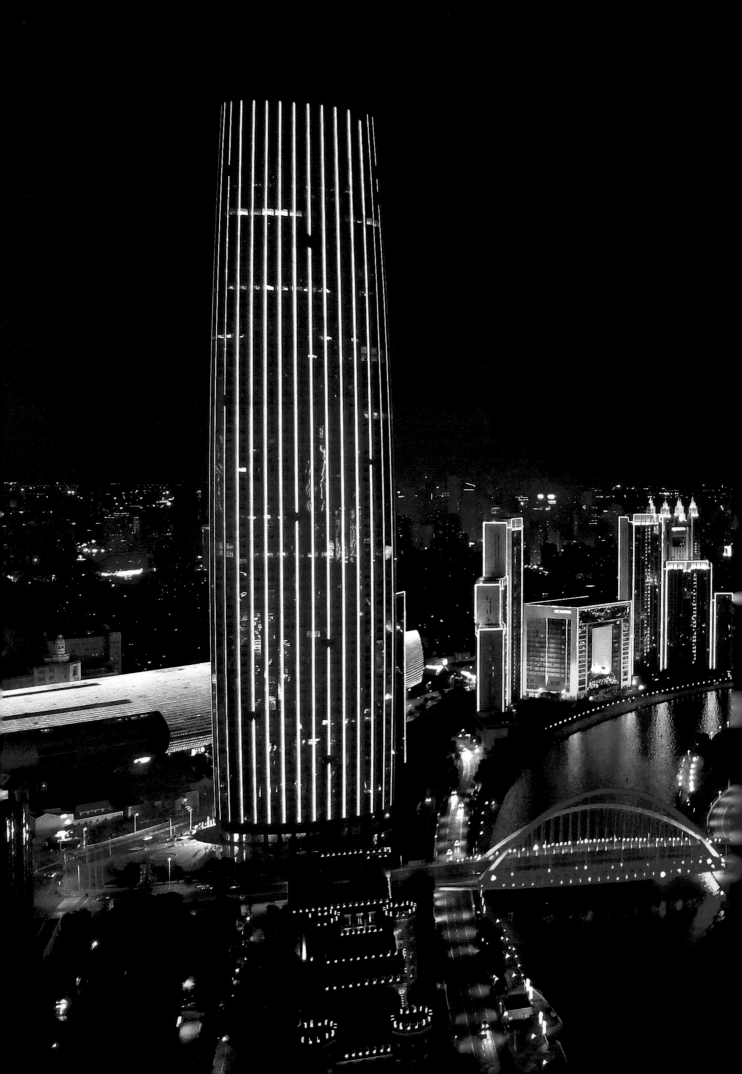

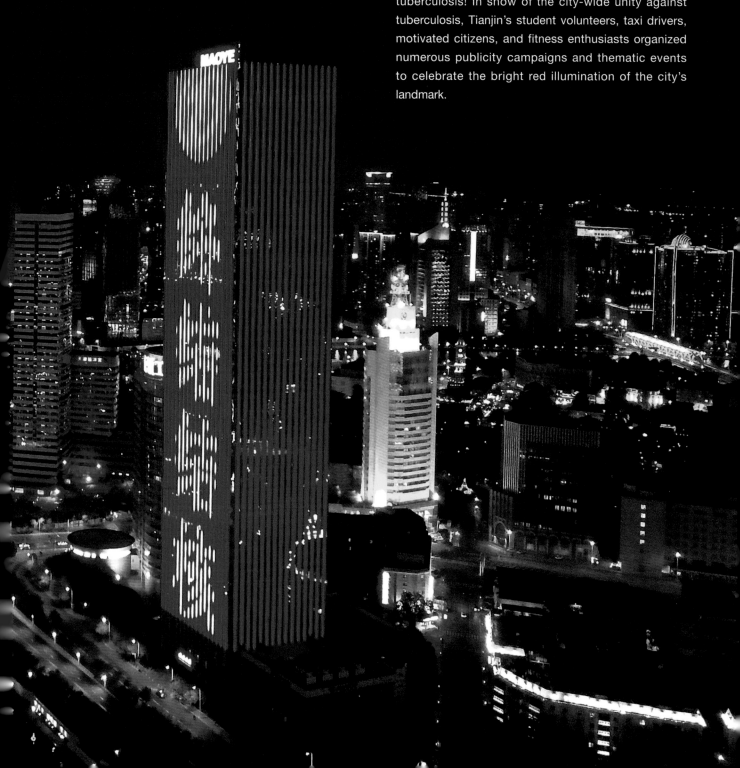

天津
Tianjin

茂业大厦是天津城市中心的地标性建筑，它的红色诠释的是攻克和战胜结核病的强大力量！天津的学生志愿者、出租车司机、热心市民及健身爱好者等积极踊跃地通过各种方式开展主题宣传活动，与城市地标的亮红行动交相辉映，成为结核病防治而众志成城的一道风景线。

Maoye Mansion, a landmark in Tianjin's city center, lit up in red, symbolizing the strong will to prevail over tuberculosis! In show of the city-wide unity against tuberculosis, Tianjin's student volunteers, taxi drivers, motivated citizens, and fitness enthusiasts organized numerous publicity campaigns and thematic events to celebrate the bright red illumination of the city's landmark.

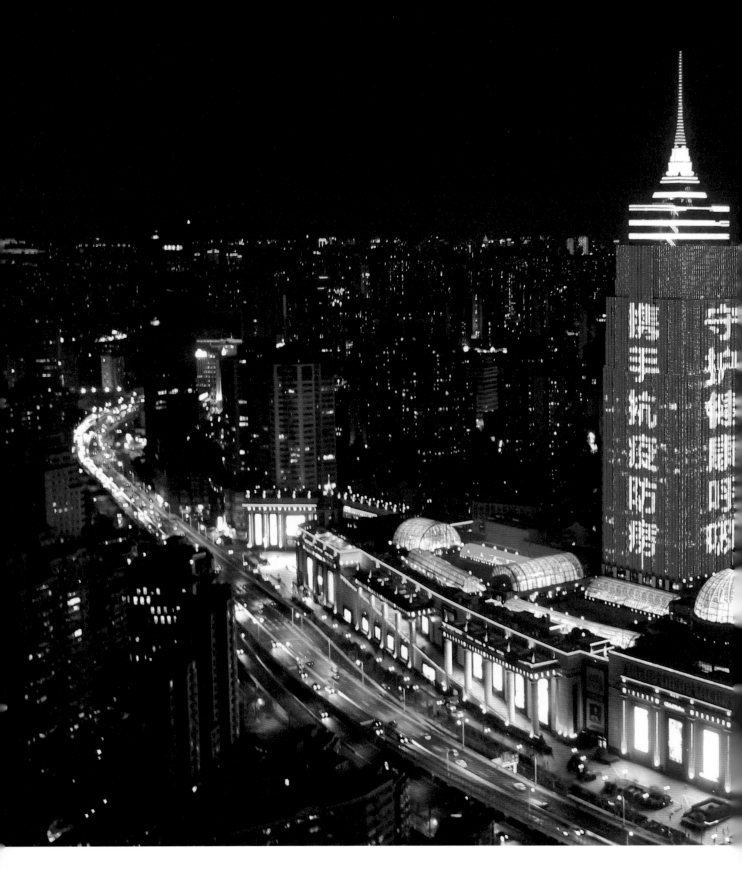

上海

Shanghai

上海环球港是全球中心城区最大的购物中心之一，空中屋顶花园瑰丽绽放、周边交通枢纽忙碌繁华，这里成为抗击结核病的宣传阵营！

The Global Harbor in Shanghai, one of the biggest shopping complexes in the downtown area, has a beautiful rooftop garden and sits in the hustle and bustle of the high streets. It becomes a beacon of publicity in the fight against tuberculosis.

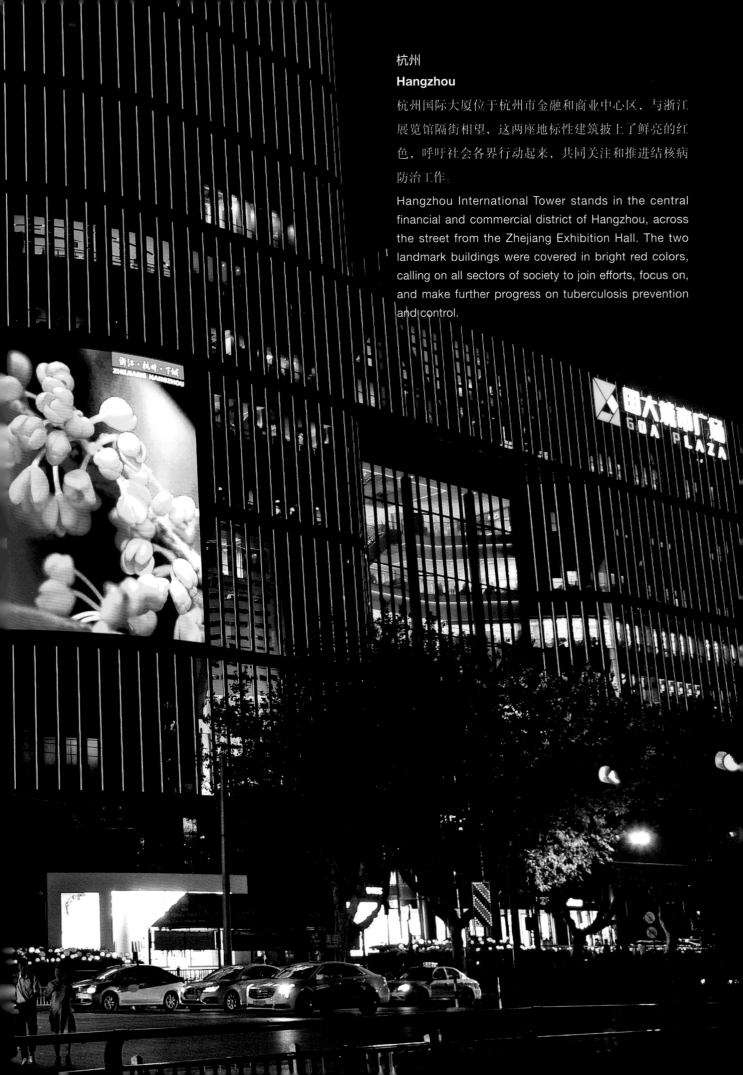

杭州

Hangzhou

杭州国际大厦位于杭州市金融和商业中心区，与浙江展览馆隔街相望，这两座地标性建筑披上了鲜亮的红色，呼吁社会各界行动起来，共同关注和推进结核病防治工作。

Hangzhou International Tower stands in the central financial and commercial district of Hangzhou, across the street from the Zhejiang Exhibition Hall. The two landmark buildings were covered in bright red colors, calling on all sectors of society to join efforts, focus on, and make further progress on tuberculosis prevention and control.

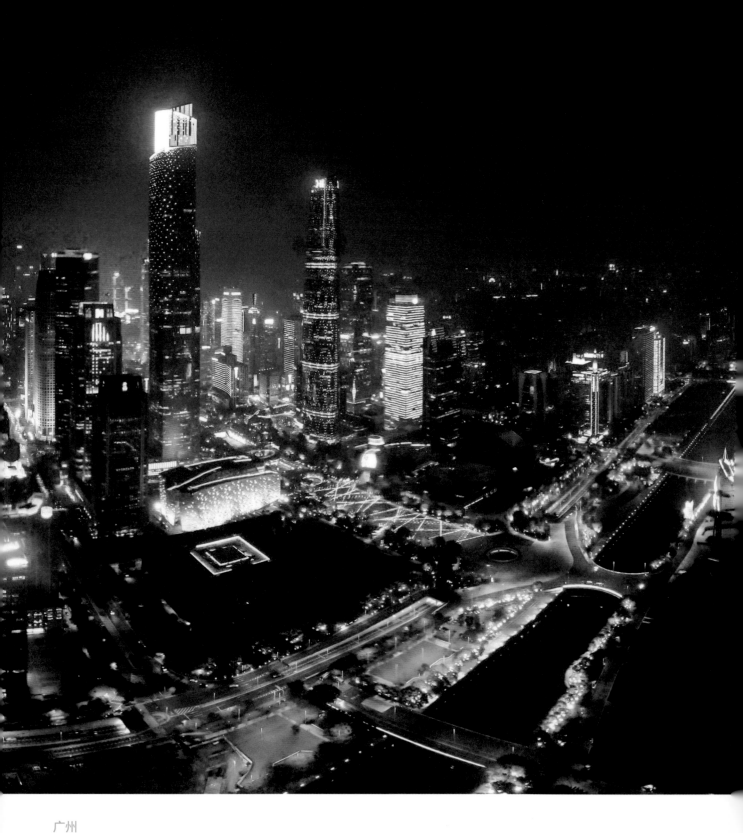

广州

Guangzhou

广州塔昵称"小蛮腰",是中国第一、世界第三的旅游观光塔,向世人展示腾飞广州、挑战自我、面向世界的视野和气魄。终止结核病这项新使命赋予了它别样的色彩和美丽!

The Canton Tower, also known as the Slim Waist for its shape, is China's top and the world's third most famous sightseeing tower. It symbolizes the bold vision and ambition of Guangzhou to take off, embrace the world, and push limits. The new mission to end TB gave it a different color and charisma!

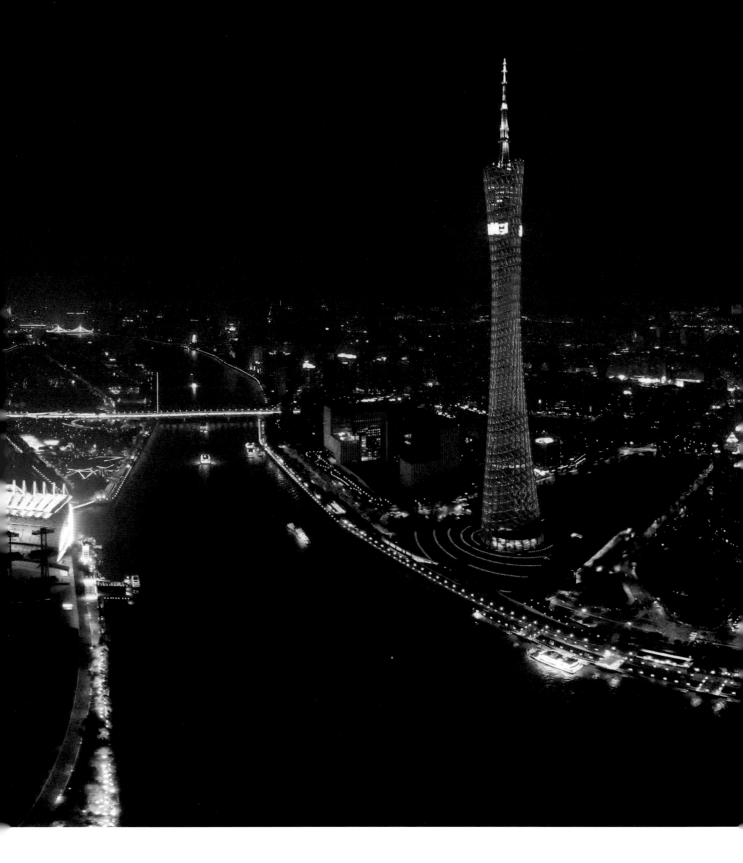

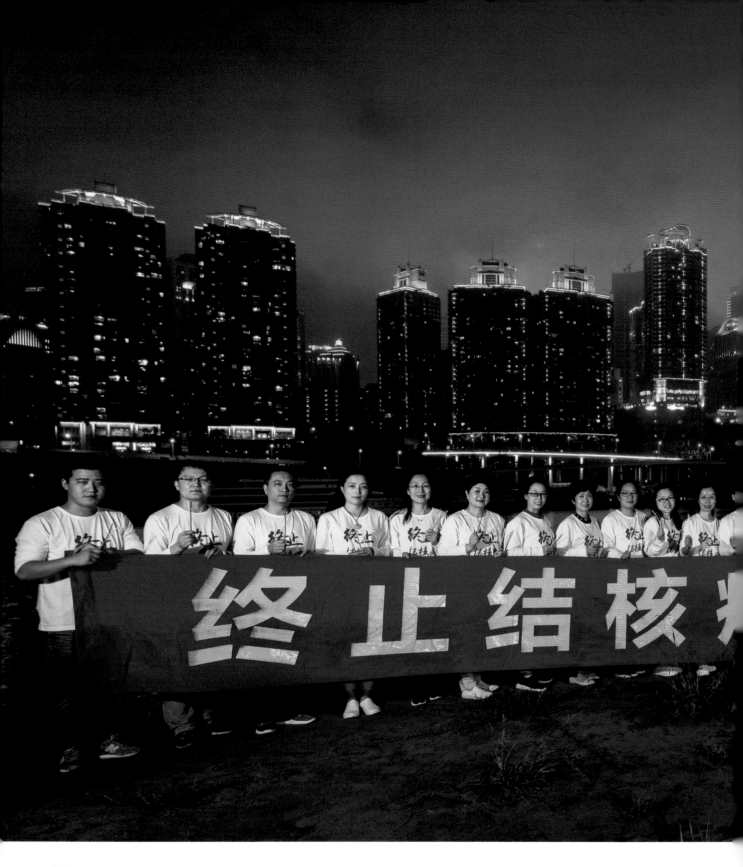

重庆

Chongqing

重庆菜园坝长江大桥是中国第二大跨度拱桥，它的建成曾创下三项世界第一，是目前国内最大的公共交通和城市轻轨两用大跨径拱桥，它亮起了旗帜性的中国红。

The Caiyuanba Yangtze River Bridge in Chongqing is China's second longest arch bridge whose award-winning design has won three world records. This dual-use road-rail arch bridge currently hosts six lanes of traffic and two tracks of light rail. It lit up in the iconic Chinese red.

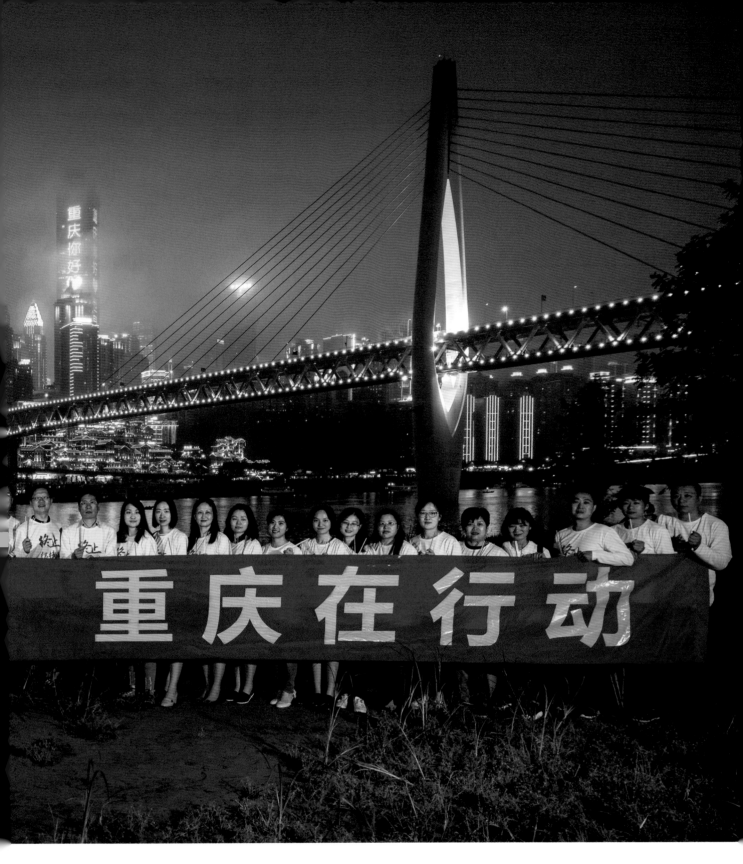

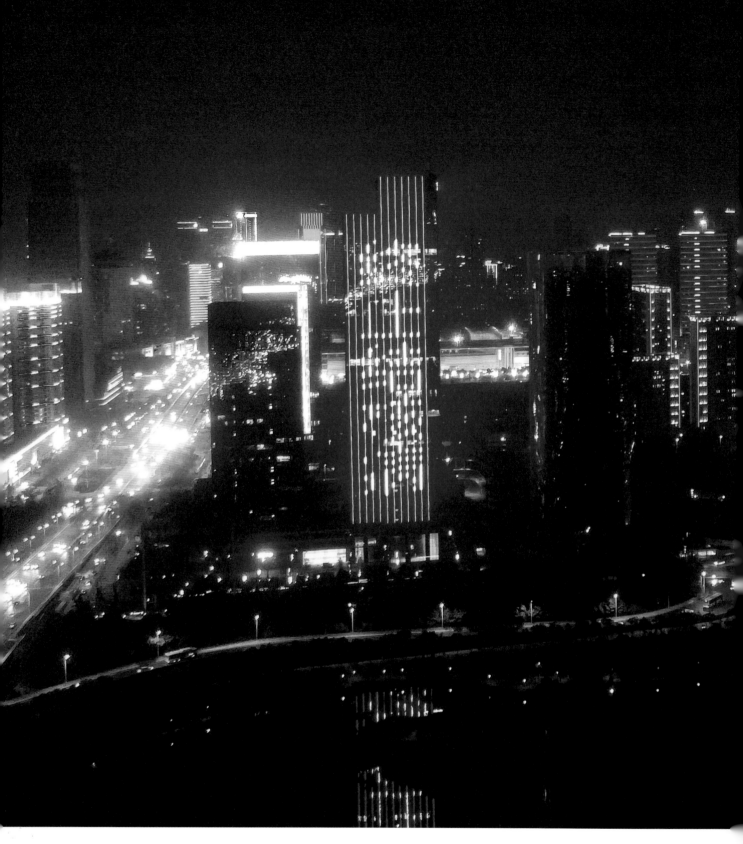

武汉

Wuhan

武汉市是中国长江、汉水交汇之处的一颗璀璨明珠，绵延25公里的两江四岸，1 000多座地标性建筑同时"披"上一抹鲜亮的红色。因为一种病，点亮一座城，是我们为终止结核病做出的庄严承诺。

Wuhan City is a bright pearl at the intersection of the Yangtze River and Hanshul River in China. About 25 kilometers across the two rivers and four banks, more than 1,000 landmarks were covered the bright red color. Lighting up a city for one disease is our solemn commitment to end TB.

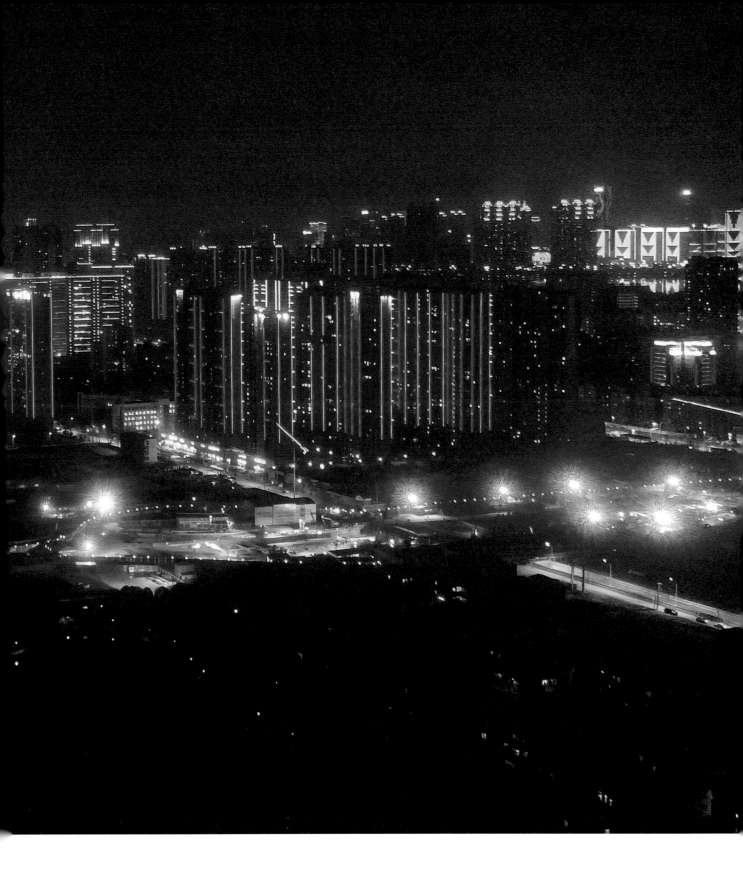

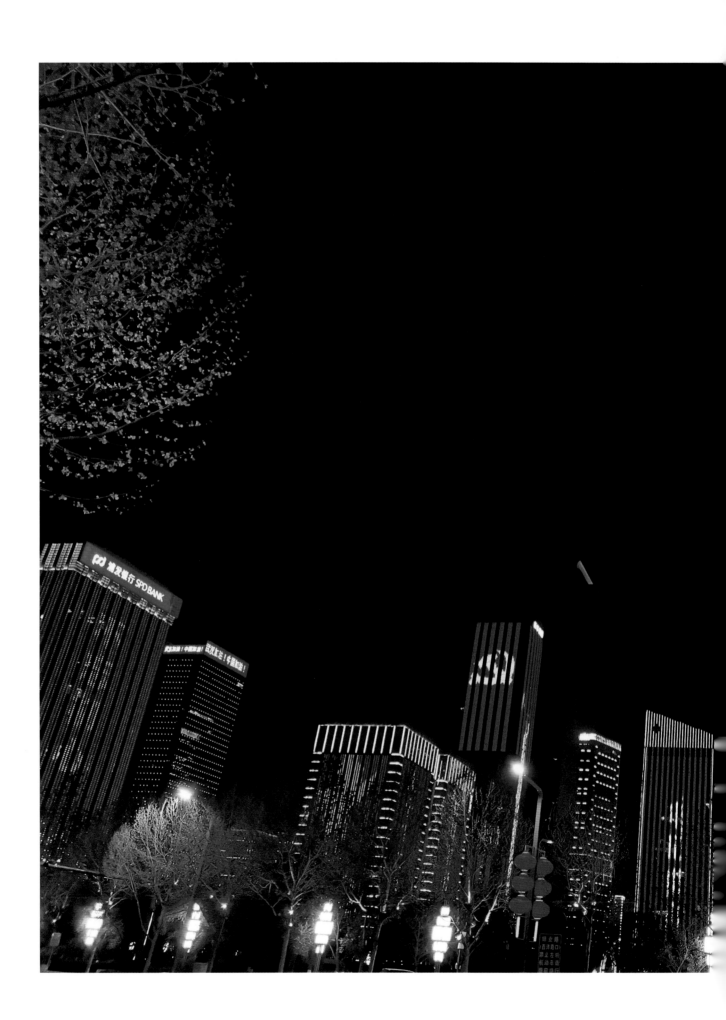

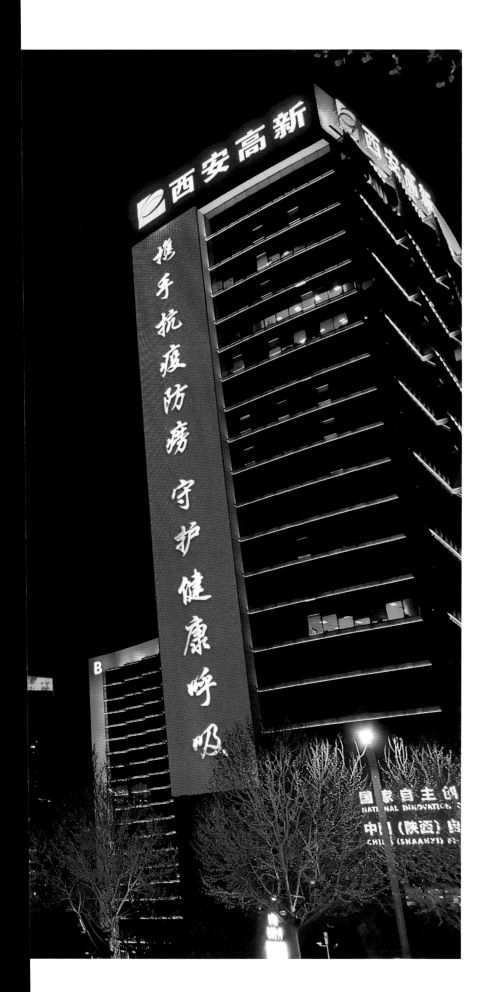

西安

Xi'an

西安都市之门是西安市的地标建筑，一抹抹的"长安"红，在夜幕下璀璨绽放，表达了古城人民遏制结核病的决心和力量！

The City Gate, landmark building in the ancient city of Xi'an, decorated with the red lights, shining brightly in the night, shows the determination and strength of the people to stop TB!

公益大使
春风化雨

Chapter 8

Significant Impact
of the Goodwill
Ambassador

让老百姓认识结核病的危害，普及结核病防治知识，倡导消除歧视，提振抗击结核病的信心，需要动员全社会共同参与。公众人物通过自身的号召力影响着越来越多的人关注结核病，鼓舞着越来越多的人走上防治结核病的公益之路。

It takes the mobilization of society-wide participation to raise public awareness about the dangers of tuberculosis, popularize the knowledge of tuberculosis prevention and treatment, advocate against discrimination, and boost the confidence in the fight against tuberculosis. Through their convening power, public figures are calling for increased attention to tuberculosis and inspiring others to join in the public health effort to end tuberculosis.

2007, 浙江义乌　　2007, Yiwu, Zhejiang

2007年，我国著名歌唱家彭丽媛成为首位全国结核病防治形象大使。十多年来，她初心不改，认真履职，拍摄公益广告和宣传海报，参加宣传倡导活动，慰问基层医务人员，探望结核病患者及其亲属。从城市到乡村、从校园到建筑工地、从医院到患者家中。她的足迹遍布中国的众多角落，被结核病防治战线的工作者和志愿者们亲切地称为"彭大使"。

In 2007, a renowned singer from China, Madame PENG Liyuan, became the first national ambassador for tuberculosis prevention and control. For more than a decade, she has stayed true to this mission and faithfully discharged her duties, by appearing in public service advertisements and posters, participating in advocacy and awareness campaigns, visiting grassroots medical personnel, patients and their families. She has graced the four corners of the country and beyond, from urban to rural areas, from school campuses to construction sites, from hospitals to patients' homes, from earthquake-stricken areas to international forums. For her relentless effort, Madame PENG has been addressed by the health professionals and volunteers working on the frontline of tuberculosis prevention as Ambassador PENG.

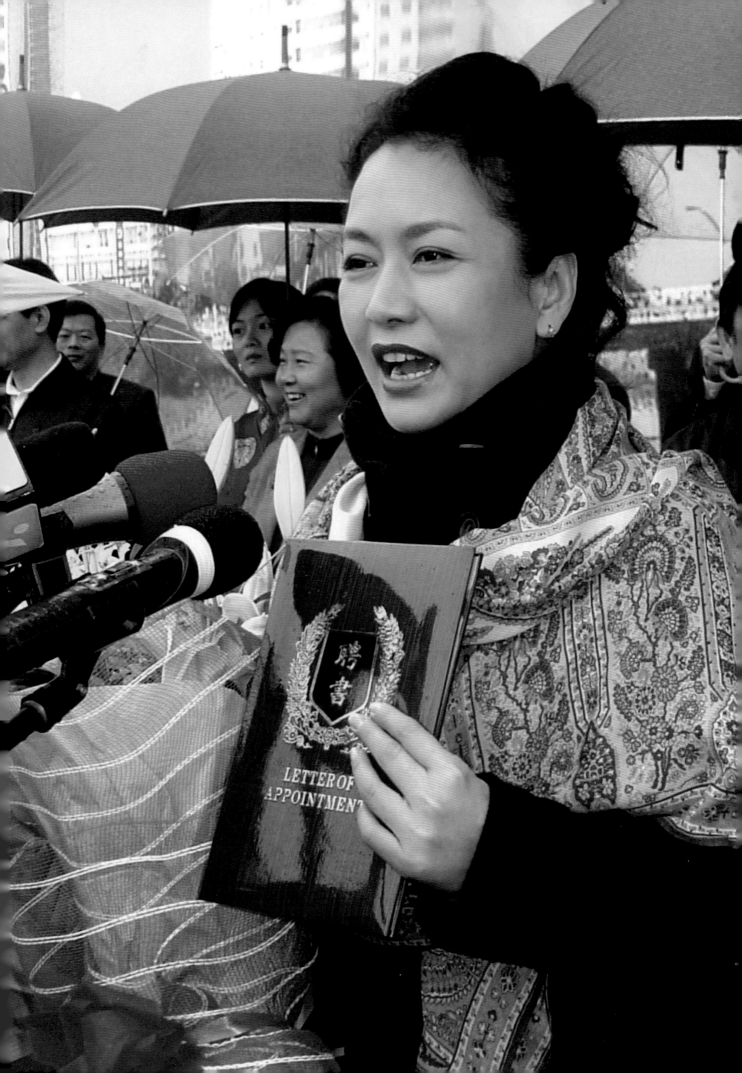

2008年，四川汶川发生特大地震灾难，彭丽媛和卫生部一行赶赴都江堰灾区捐赠结核病防治设备。在安置点举行的结核病防治健康宣传义诊活动上，彭大使走上舞台向在场群众宣传结核病防治核心知识。在围观乡亲们的强烈要求下，她演唱了一首《父老乡亲》，道出了对灾区百姓的不尽情谊。很多人都感动得流下了眼泪，彭大使递给他们的宣传册，乡亲们都一直珍藏着。

In 2008, in the immediate aftermath of the Wenchuan earthquake in Sichuan province, Madame PENG Liyuan and officials of the Ministry of Health arrived at the disaster-stricken area of Dujiangyan to donate TB prevention and control equipment. While attending an event to raise TB prevention and control awareness and provide free medical consultation at the resettlement site, Madame PENG took to the stage to give out essential information about tuberculosis prevention and control, and at the passionate prompting of the audience, she performed the song To My Folks to show that her heart was with the people affected by the disaster. Many were moved to tears by the song and have kept the brochure Madame PENG handed to them till this day.

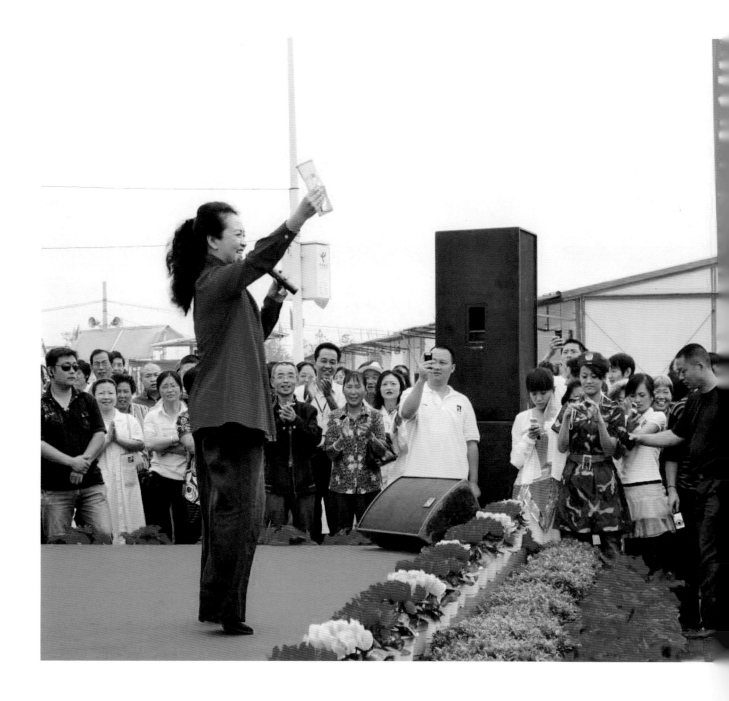

2008年　四川都江堰　　2008, Dujiangyan, Sichuan

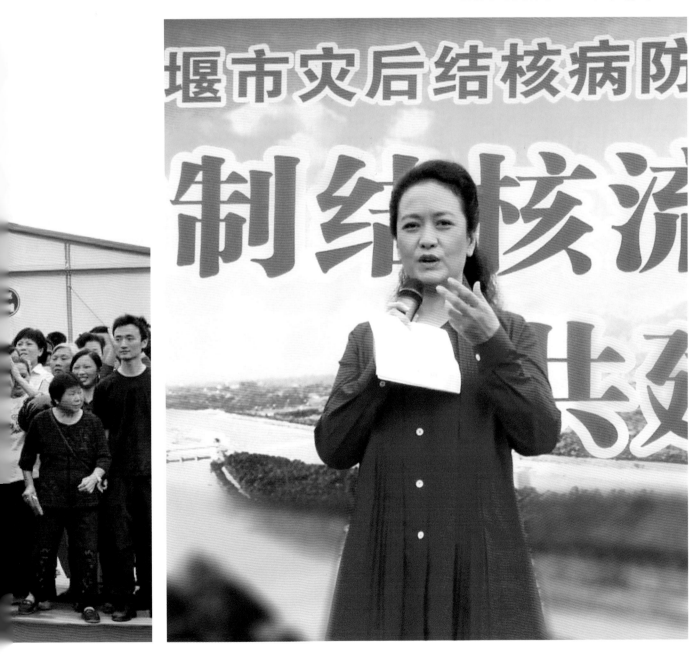

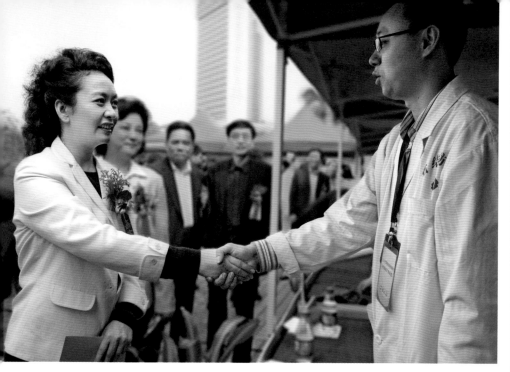

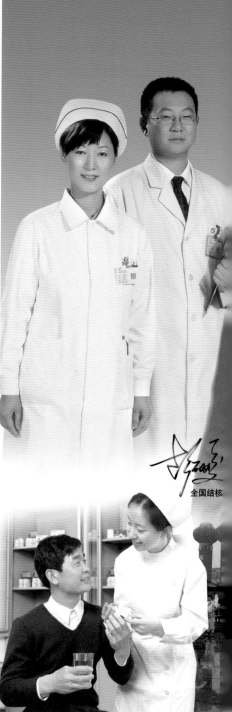

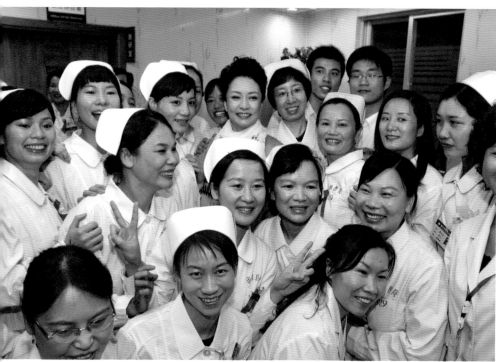

全国结核

2009年　广东东莞　　2009, Dongguan, Guangdong
2010年　广西南宁　　2010, Nanning, Guangxi

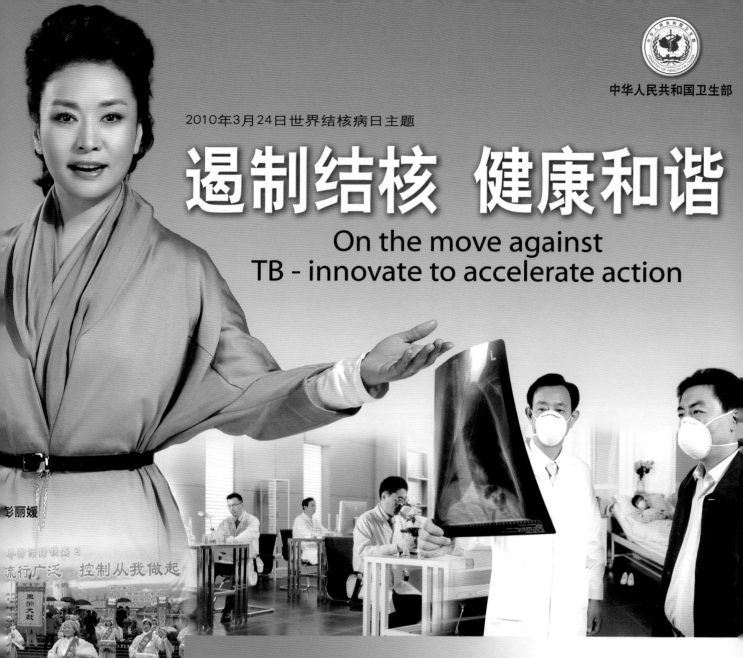

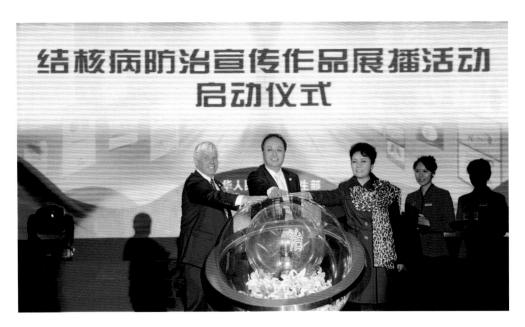

2011年　北京　　2011, Beijing

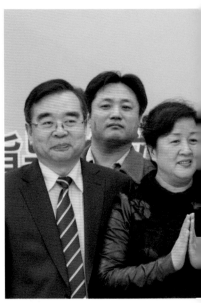

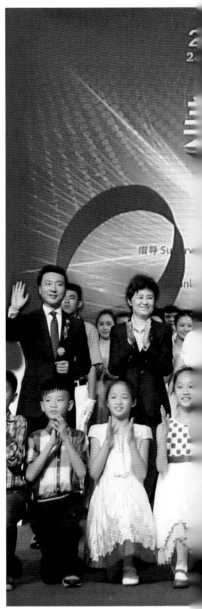

2014年　北京　　2014, Beijing

2015年　海南海口　　2015, Haikou, Hainan

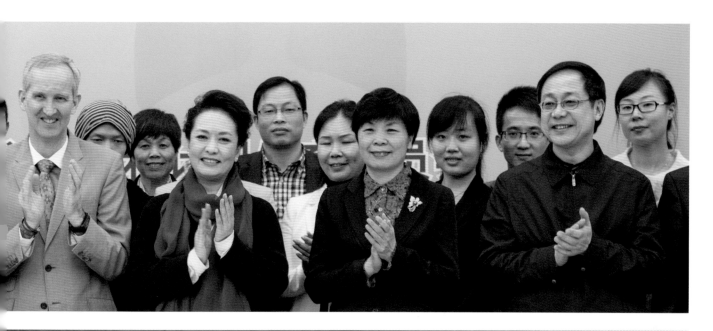

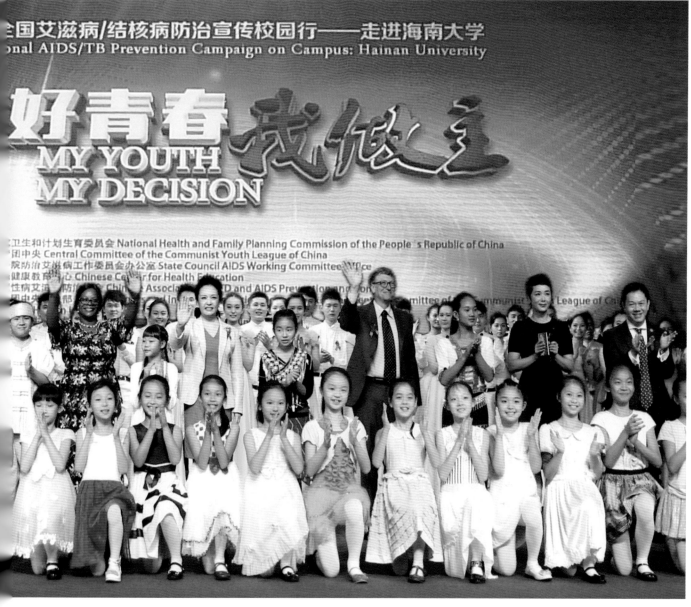

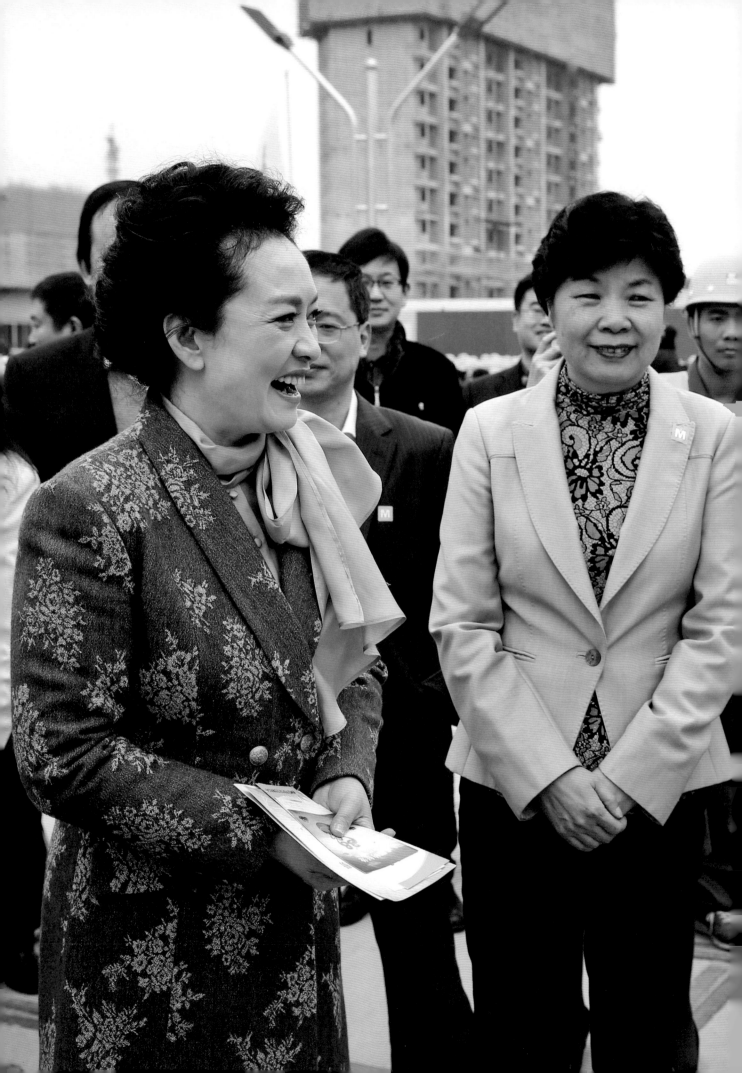

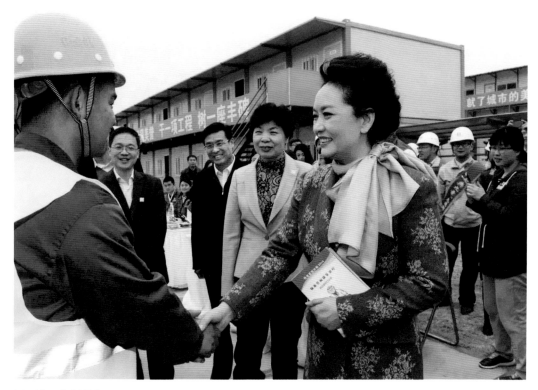

2016年　北京通州　2016, Tongzhou, Beijing

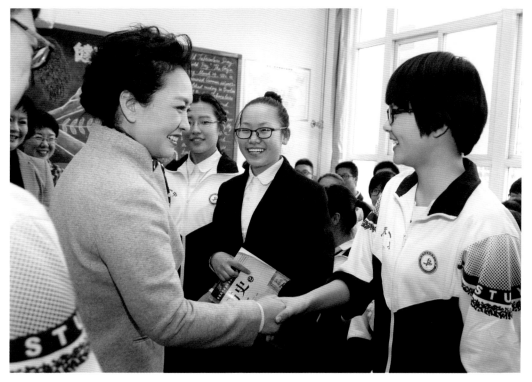

2017年　天津宝坻　2017, Baodi, Tianjin

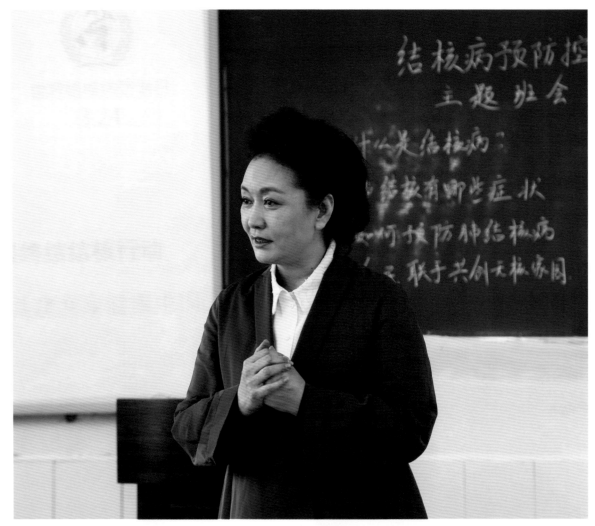

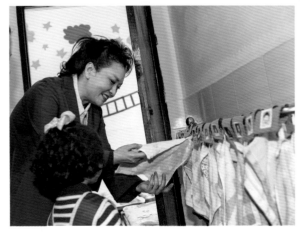

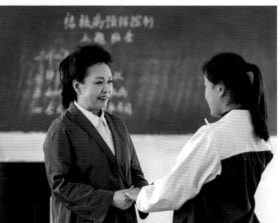

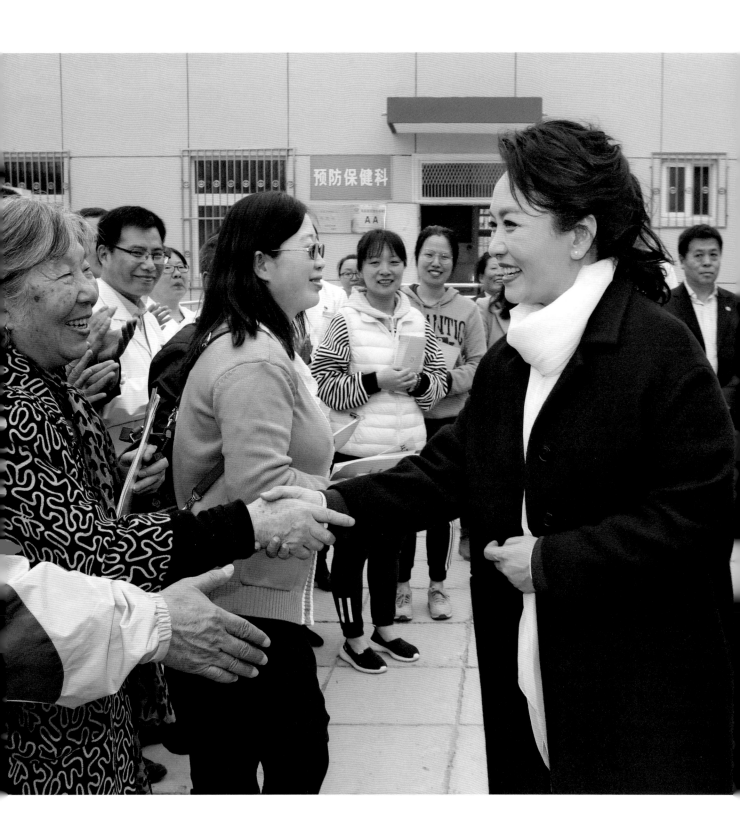

2019年　北京昌平　　2019, Changping, Beijing

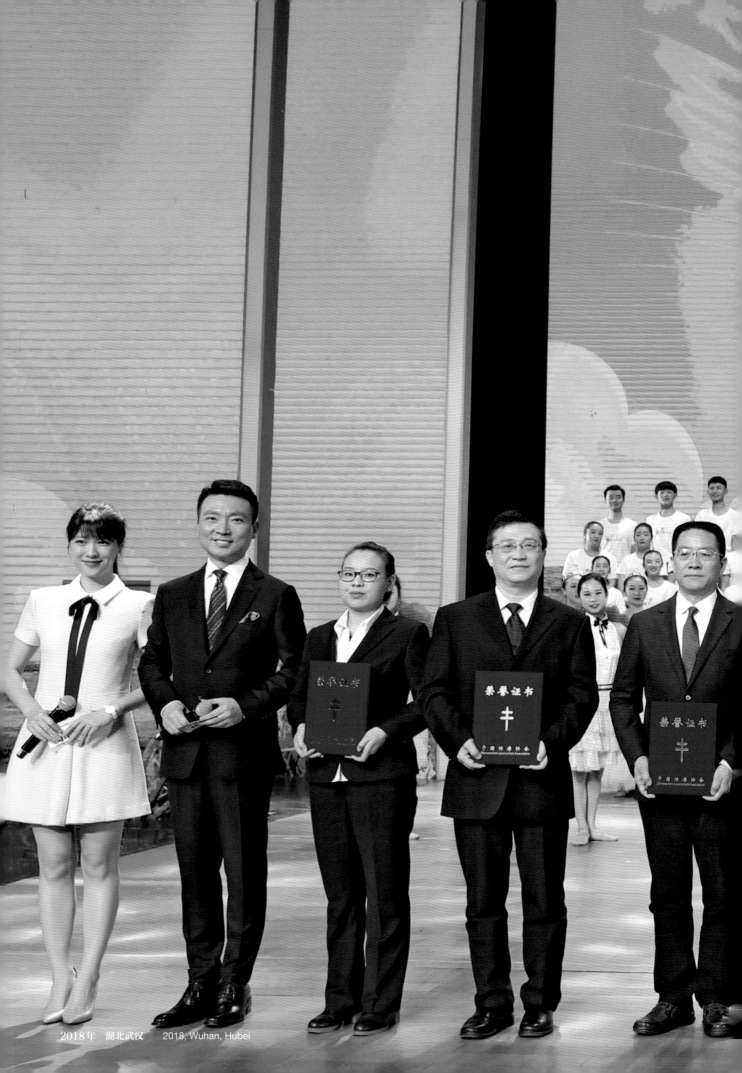

2018年　湖北武汉　2018, Wuhan, Hubei

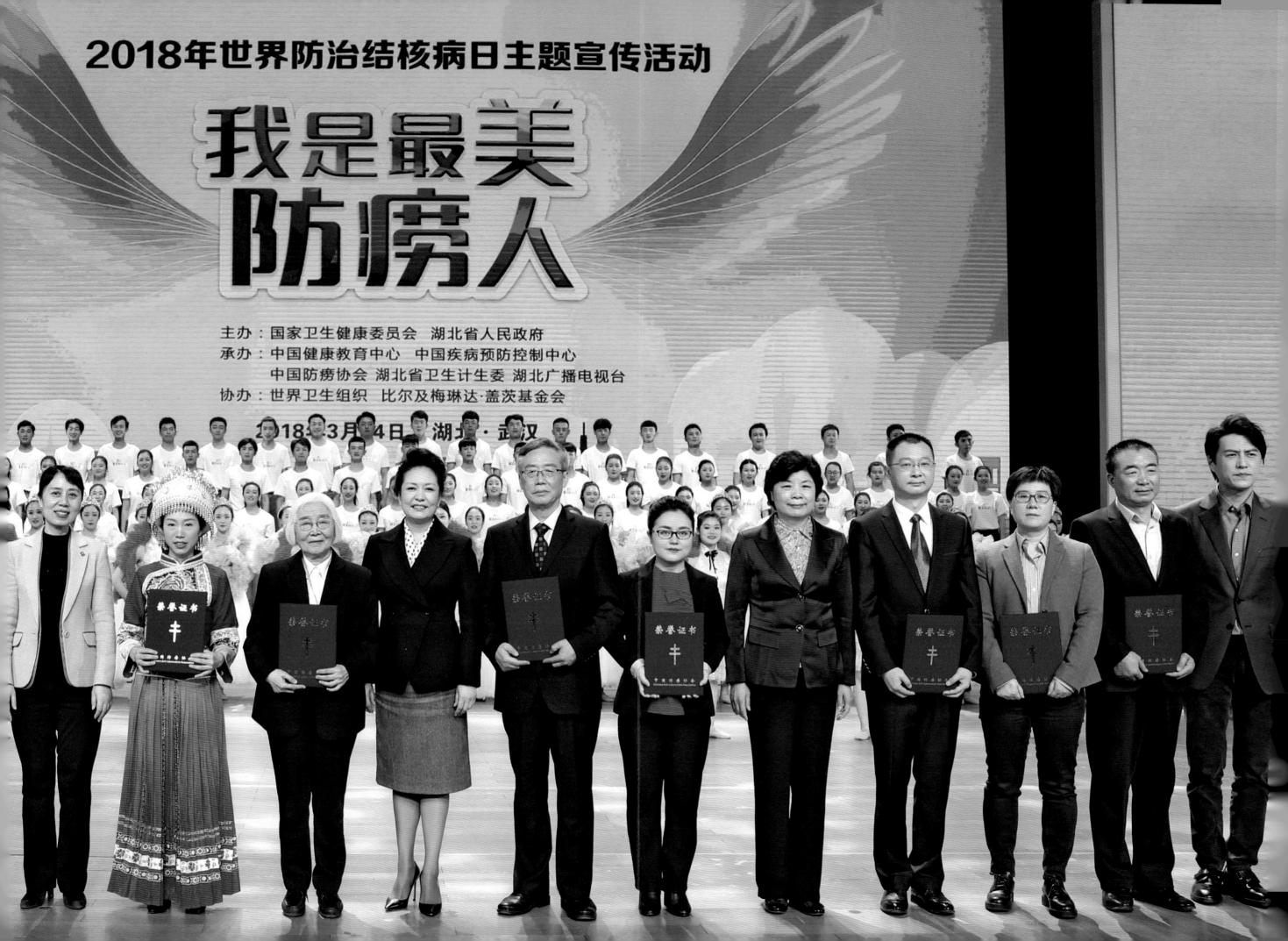

2018年世界防治结核病日主题宣传活动

我是最美
防痨人

主办：国家卫生健康委员会　湖北省人民政府
承办：中国健康教育中心　中国疾病预防控制中心
中国防痨协会　湖北省卫生计生委　湖北广播电视台
协办：世界卫生组织　比尔及梅琳达·盖茨基金会

2018年3月24日 湖北·武汉

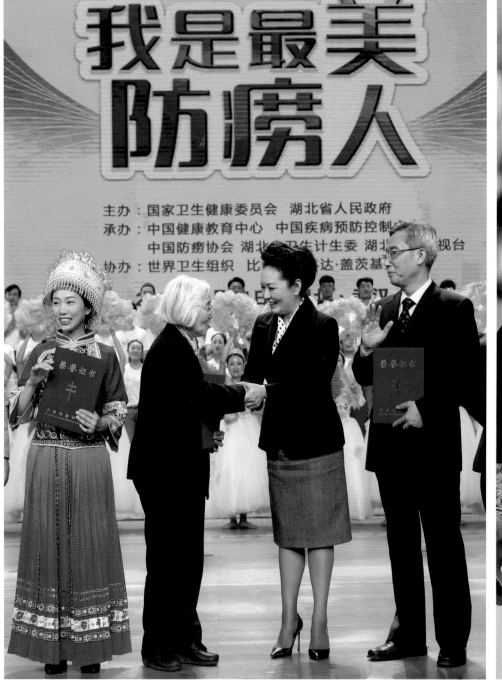

2018年 湖北武汉 2018, Wuhan, Hubei

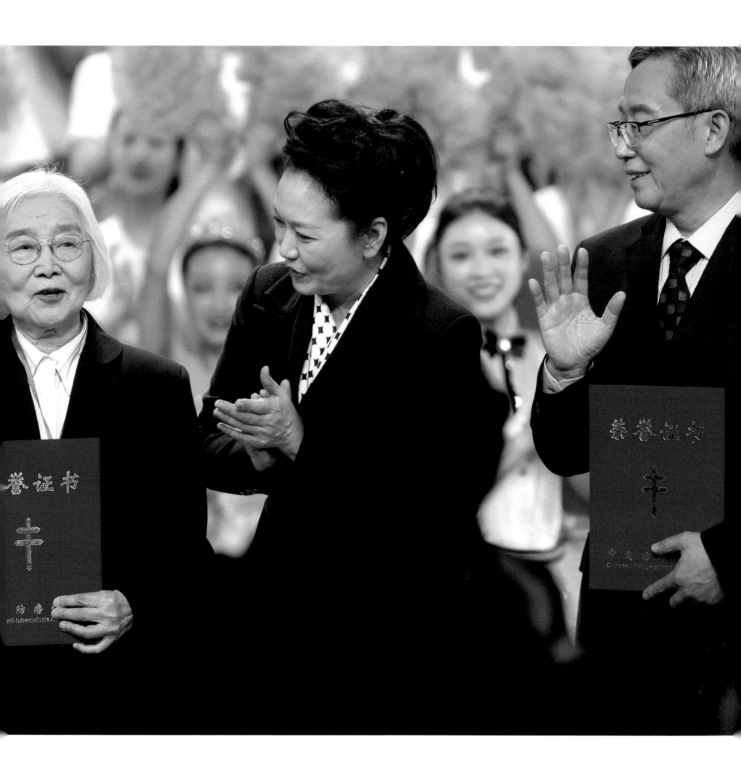

由于彭丽媛在结核病、艾滋病防治宣传倡导方面的突出贡献，2011 年世界卫生组织聘请她担任结核病/艾滋病防治亲善大使。2017 年，世界卫生组织进行了亲善大使续聘，并为彭丽媛颁发了特别贡献奖章。

In 2011, the World Health Organization appointed Madame PENG Liyuan the Goodwill Ambassador for Tuberculosis and HIV/AIDS due to her outstanding contribution in raising awareness and leading advocacy on tuberculosis and HIV/AIDS prevention and control. The WHO renewed Madame PENG's ambassadorship and awarded PENG for her special contribution in 2017.

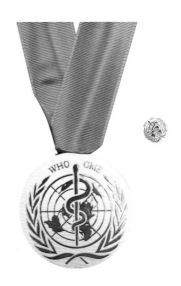

2011年　瑞士日内瓦　　2011, Geneva, Switzerland

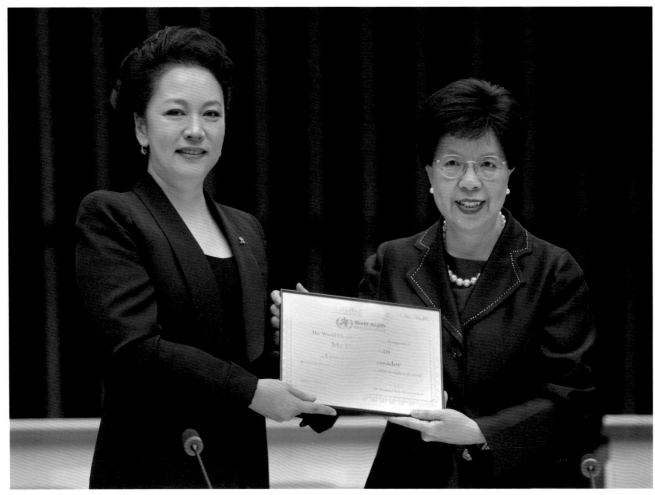

→ 2017年　瑞士日内瓦　　2017, Geneva, Switzerland

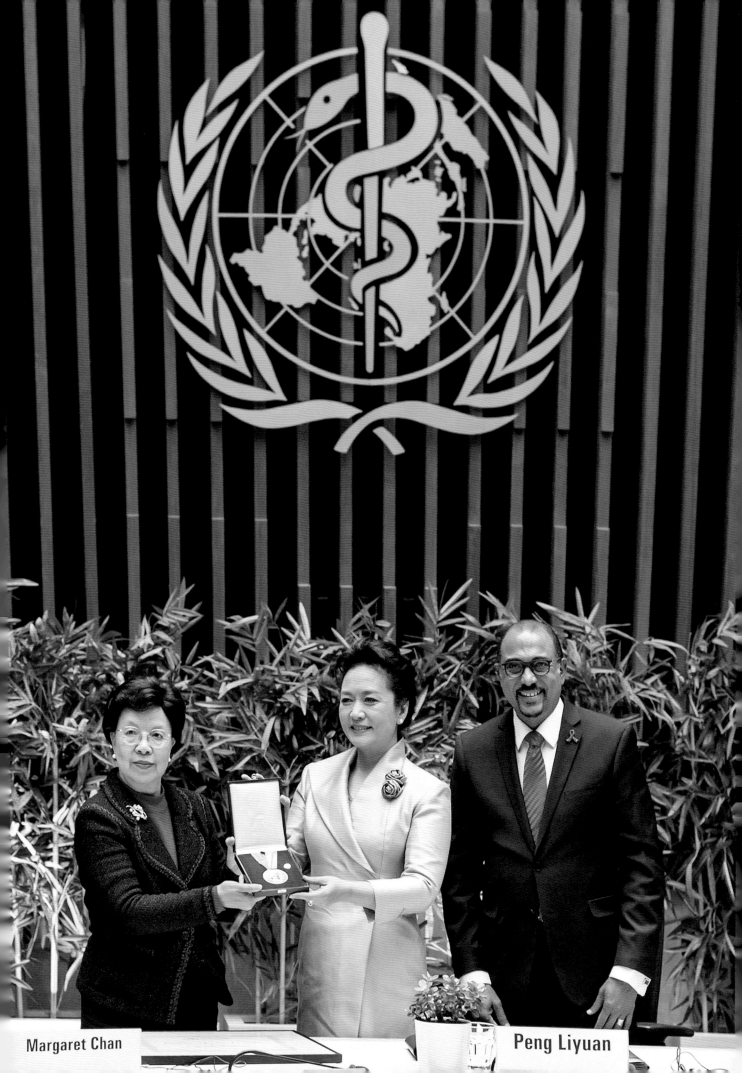

Margaret Chan   Peng Liyuan

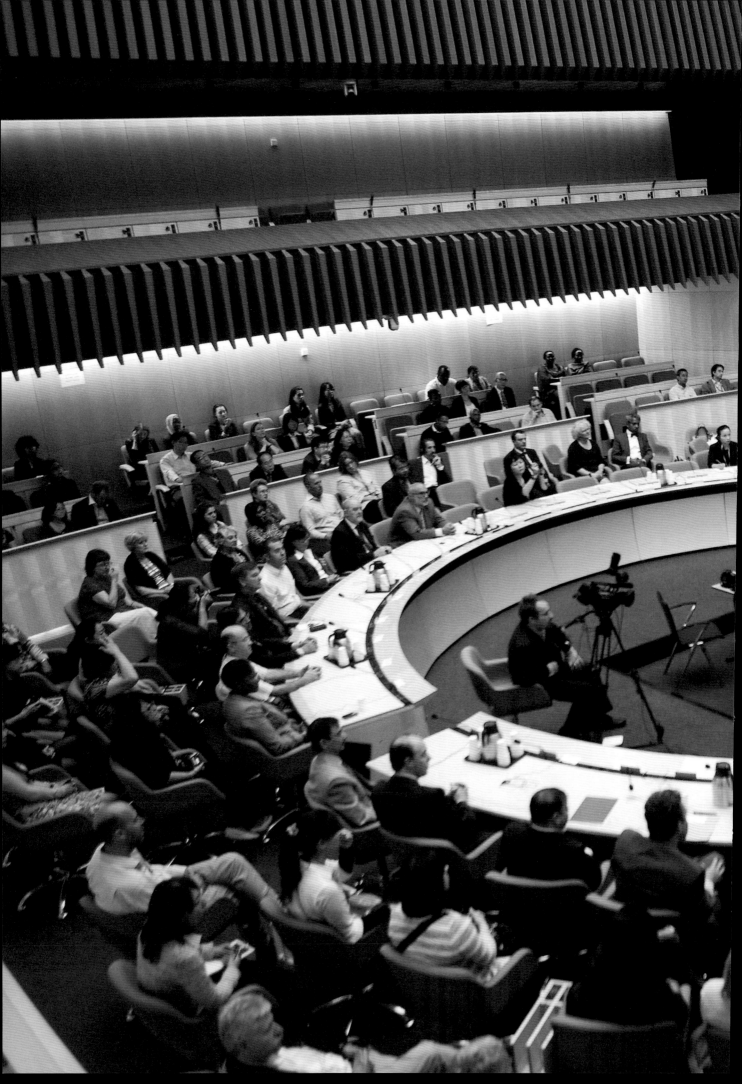

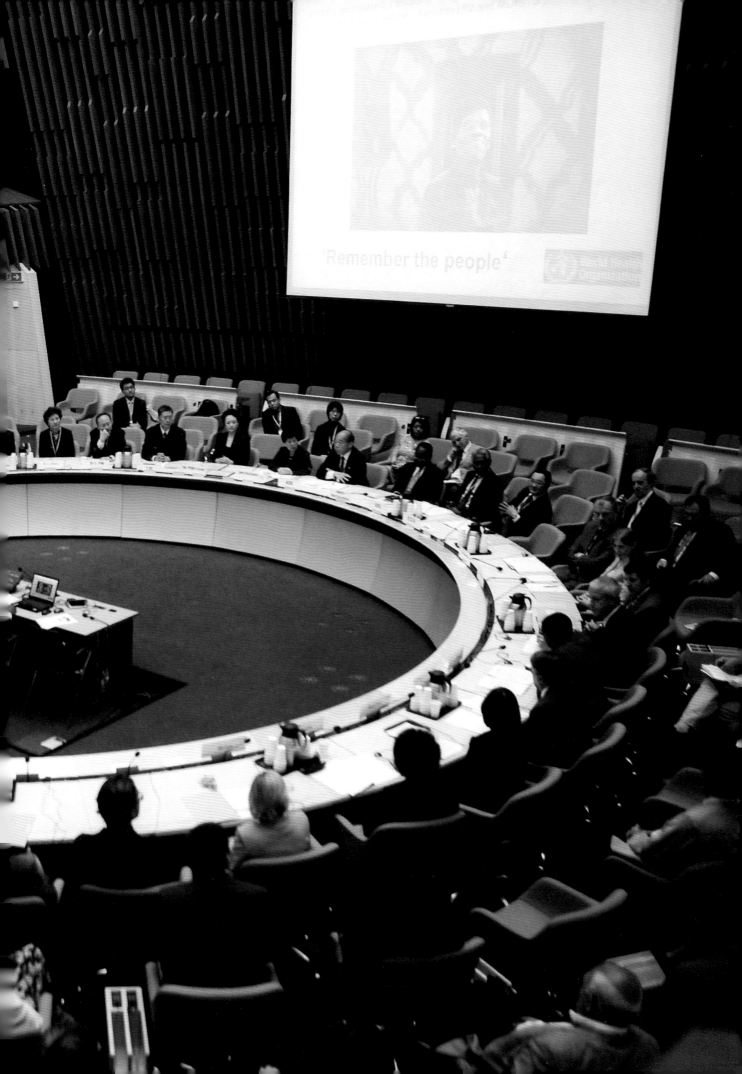

榜样的力量是无穷的，在彭丽媛大使的感召下，著名演员濮存昕、蒋雯丽、靳东、常远、马丽、中央电视台主持人白岩松、康辉、鞠萍、刚强，北京电视台主持人悦悦、刘婧等公众人物也纷纷加入了结核病防治宣传队伍。

The power of the example is infinite. Thanks to the inspirational leadership of Ambassador PENG Liyuan, famous actors and actresses such as PU Cunxin, JIANG Wenli, JIN Dong and CHANG Yuan, CCTV hosts BAI Yansong, KANG Hui, JU Ping and GANG Qiang, Beijing TV hosts YUE Yue and LIU Jing, among other public figures, also joined the fight against TB as celebrity volunteers.

他们走进建筑工地，向农民工宣传结核病防治知识，告诉他们身体是革命的本钱，健康是幸福的基础；走进演播间，拍摄结核病防治特别节目，千万观众通过节目了解结核病防治知识；走进校园，把结核病防治知识告诉中学生，健康教育要从孩子抓起；参加结核病防治宣传活动，表演结核病防治小品，鼓励百千万志愿者把知识的火种传播出去。

They visited construction sites to publicize the knowledge of tuberculosis prevention and treatment among migrant workers. They talked with the construction workers, telling them that health is their greatest asset and the foundation of happiness.
They appeared on TV on a special program for tuberculosis control, and millions of viewers tuned in to learn about tuberculosis prevention and control.
They went to school campuses to instill in kindergarten children and middle school students the knowledge of tuberculosis prevention. Health education must start at a young age. They participated in Tuberculosis Day publicity events, performed TB prevention and control stage shows, and encouraged millions of volunteers to spread the knowledge.

2016年，蒋雯丽、康辉、悦悦参加北京电视台《养生堂》世界防治结核病日特别节目录制
In 2016, JIANG Wenli, KANG Hui and YUE Yue appeared on a feature program of Yang Sheng Tang (Wellness Clinic) on World Tuberculosis Day in the studio of Beijing TV Station.

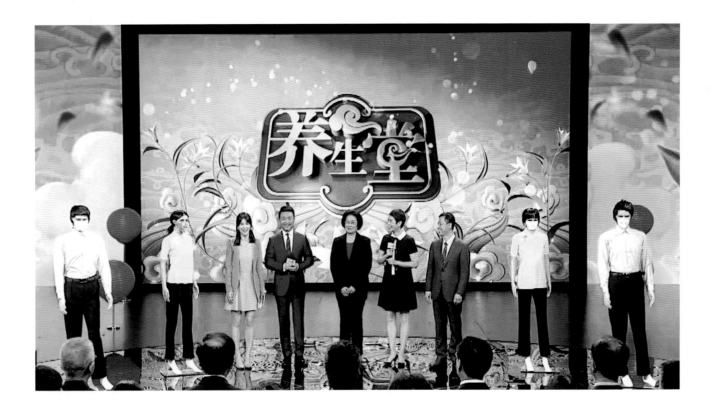

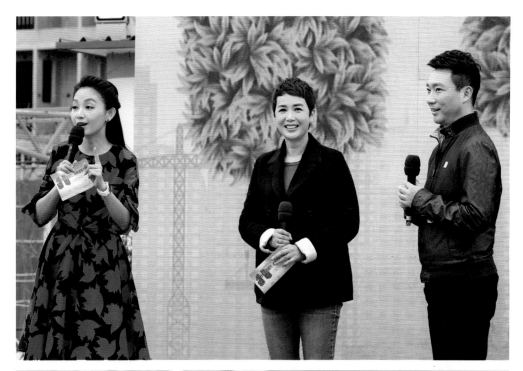

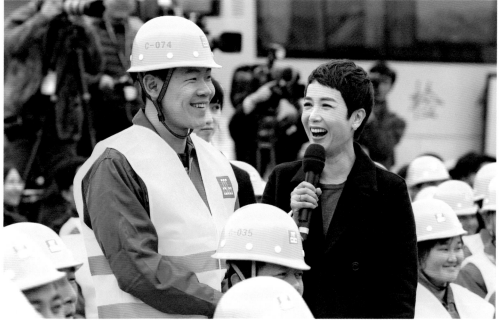

2016年，蒋雯丽、康辉、刘婧在北京通州建筑工地参加世界防治结核病日宣传活动
In 2016, JIANG Wenli, KANG Hui and LIU Jing participated in the World Tuberculosis Day publicity campaign at a construction site in Tongzhou District, Beijing.

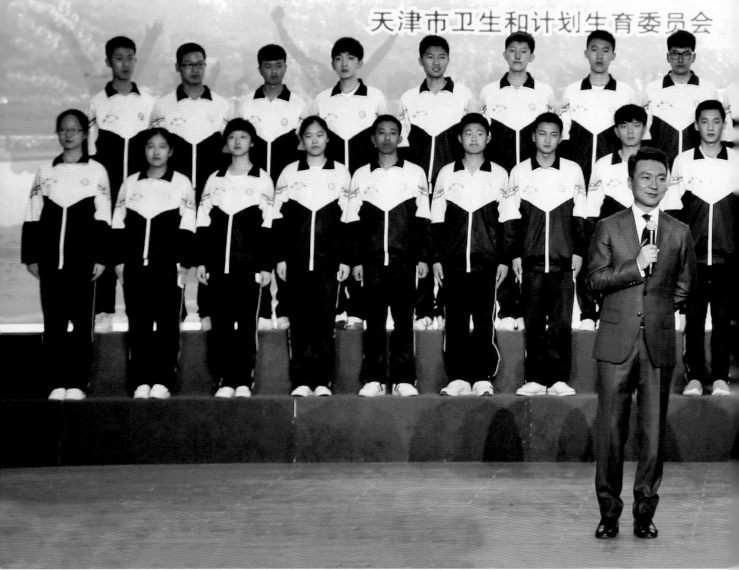

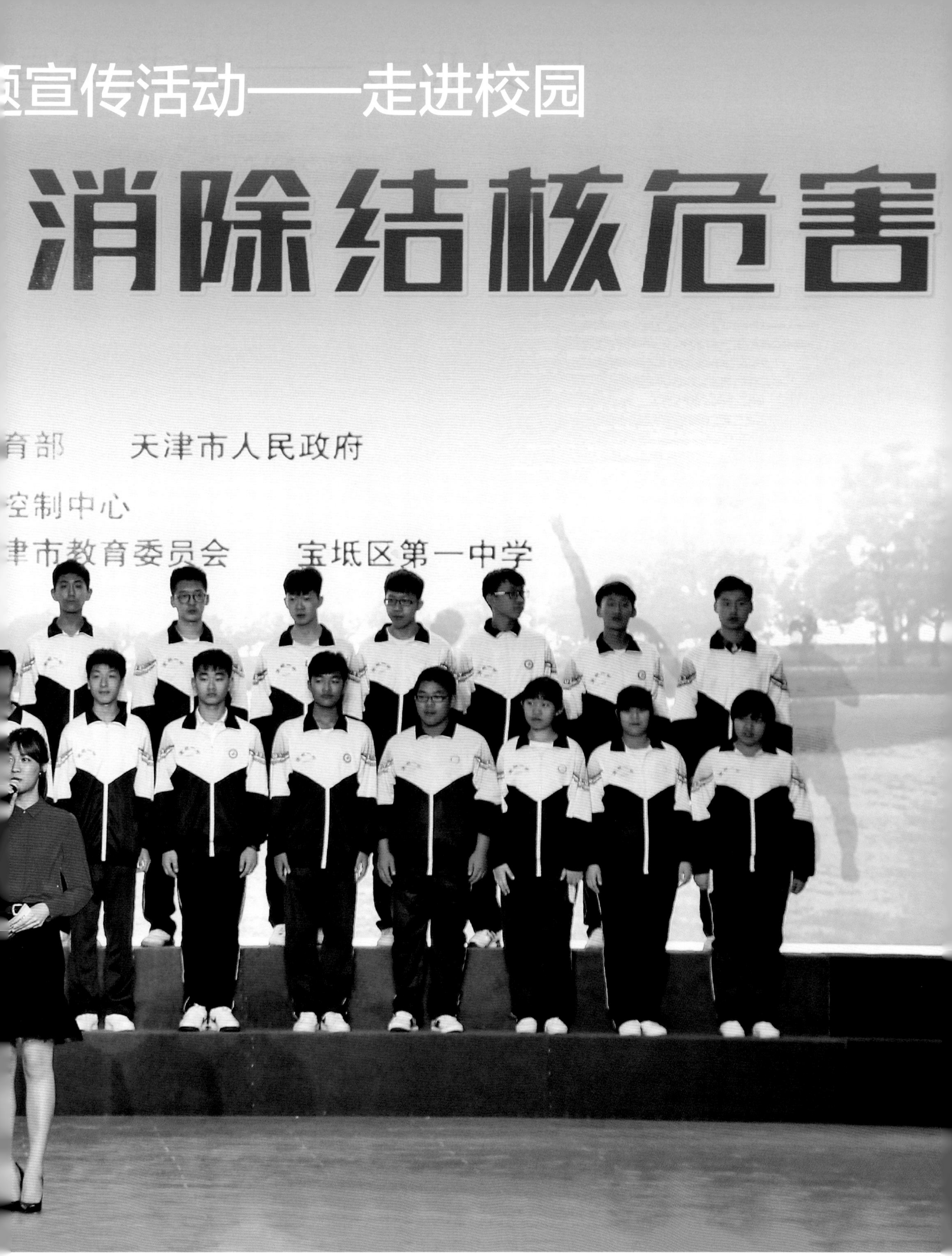

题宣传活动——走进校园

消除结核危害

育部　　　天津市人民政府

空制中心

津市教育委员会　　　宝坻区第一中学

2017年，康辉、悦悦主持校园结核病宣传活动
In 2017, KANG Hui and YUE Yue hosted a campus talk on tuberculosis control.

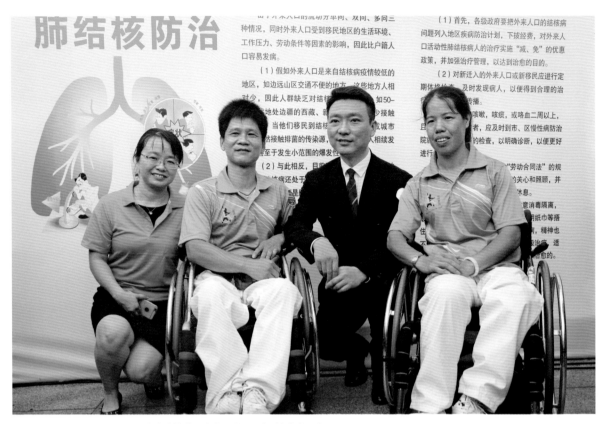

2016年，康辉在广东参加世界防治结核病日宣传活动，与志愿者们在一起
In 2016, KANG Hui participated in the World Tuberculosis Day publicity campaign in Guangdong with volunteers.

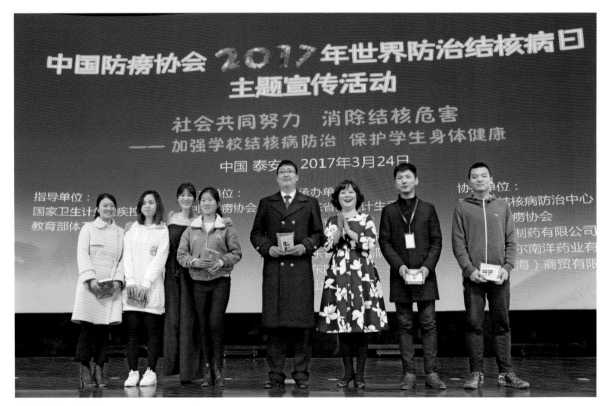

2017年，鞠萍、悦悦在山东泰安参加世界防治结核病日宣传活动，与防痨知识竞赛获奖大学生在一起
In 2017, JU Ping and YUE Yue participated in the World Tuberculosis Day publicity campaign in Tai'an, Shandong province, together with the college students that won the TB Control Knowledge Competition.

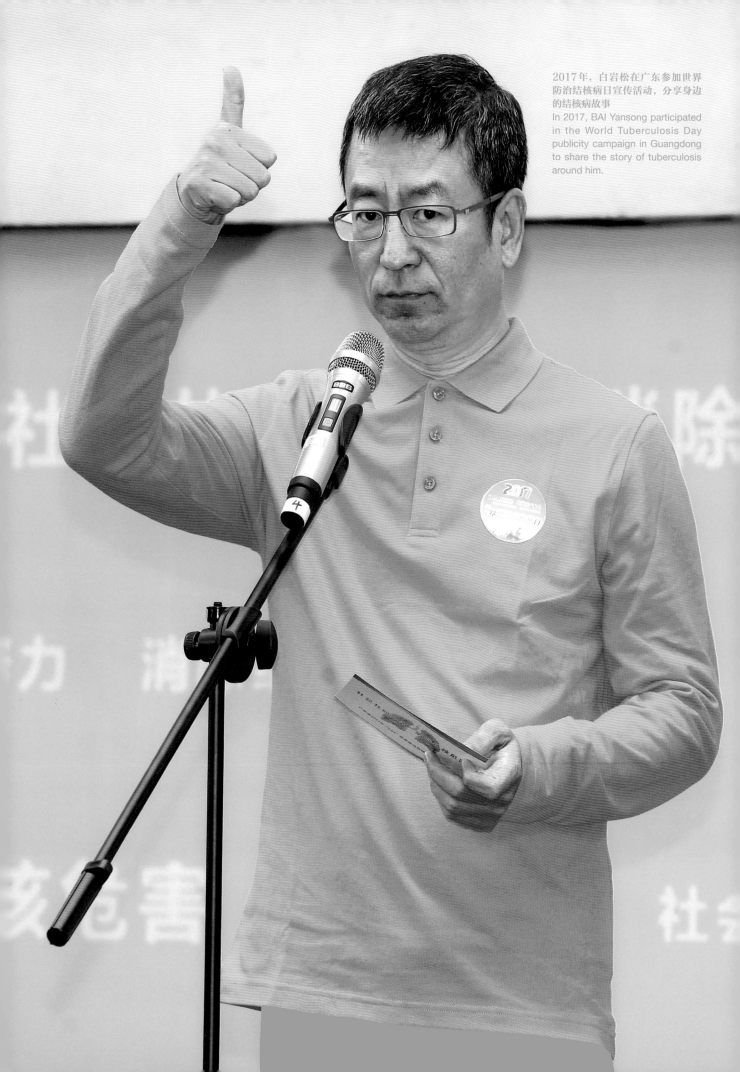

2017年，白岩松在广东参加世界防治结核病日宣传活动，分享身边的结核病故事

In 2017, BAI Yansong participated in the World Tuberculosis Day publicity campaign in Guangdong to share the story of tuberculosis around him.

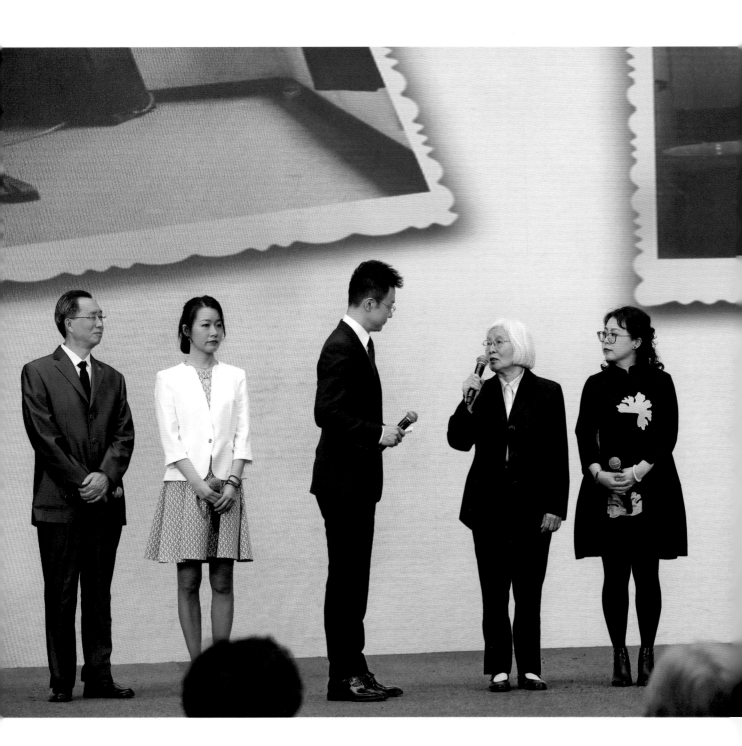

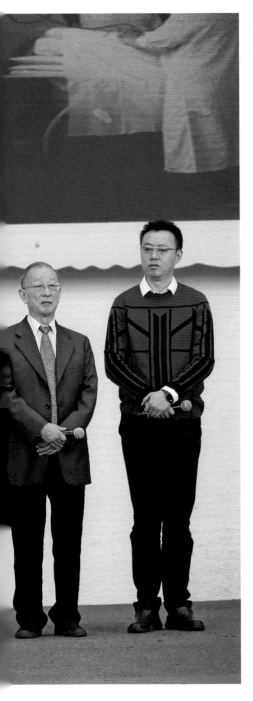

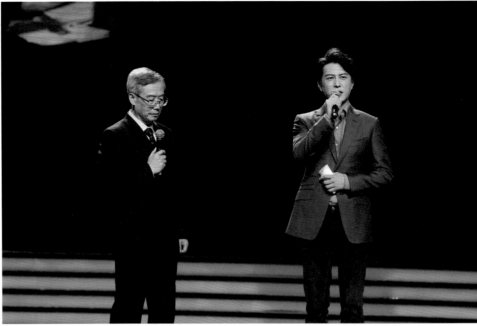

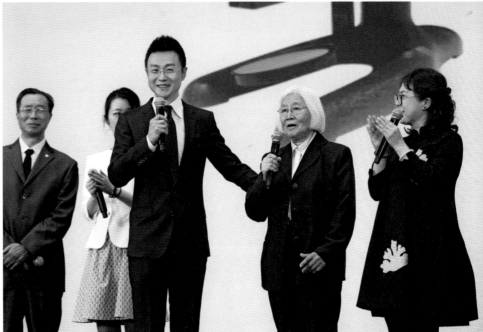

2018年，靳东参加世界防治结核病日宣传活动
In 2018, JIN Dong participated in the World Tuberculosis Day publicity campaign.

2019年，刚强主持世界防治结核病日宣传活动
In 2019, GANG Qiang hosted the World Tuberculosis Day publicity campaign.

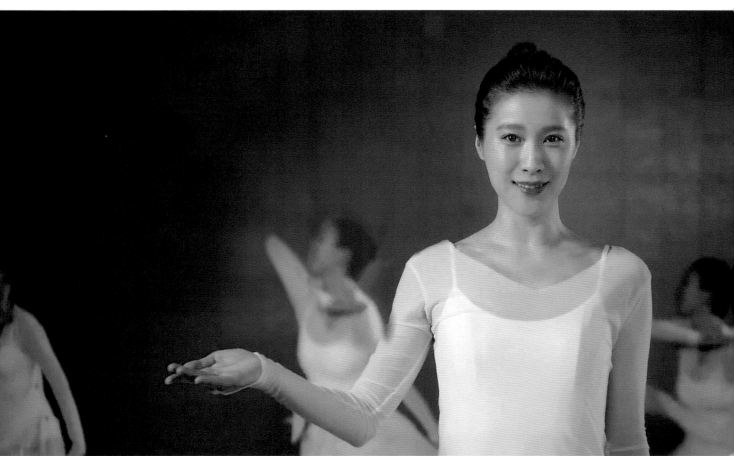

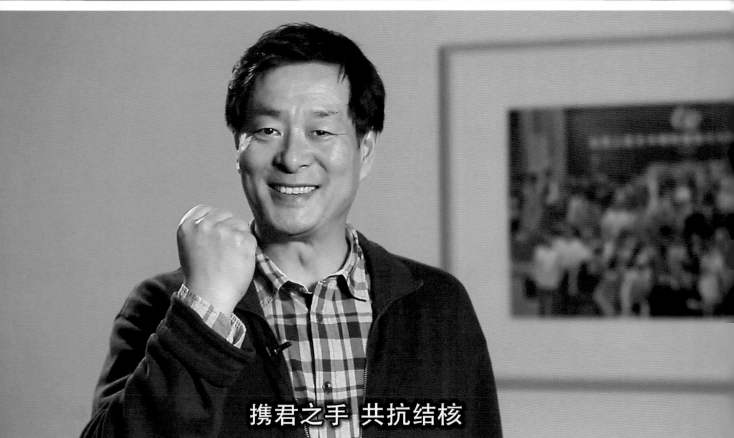

携君之手 共抗结核

濮存昕、悦悦拍摄结核病防治宣传片
Pu Cunxin and Yueyue shoot publicity video of TB prevention and control

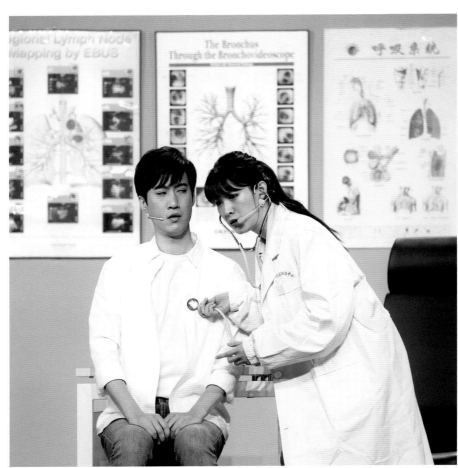

2018年，悦悦、常远表演小品《因结核而结合》
In 2018, YUE Yue, CHANG Yuan, performed stage show entitled A Match by Tuberculosis.

2019年，悦悦、常远、马丽、靳东表演小品《爱的考核》
In 2019, YUE Yue, CHANG Yuan, MA Li, and JIN Dong performed a stage drama, the Test of Love.

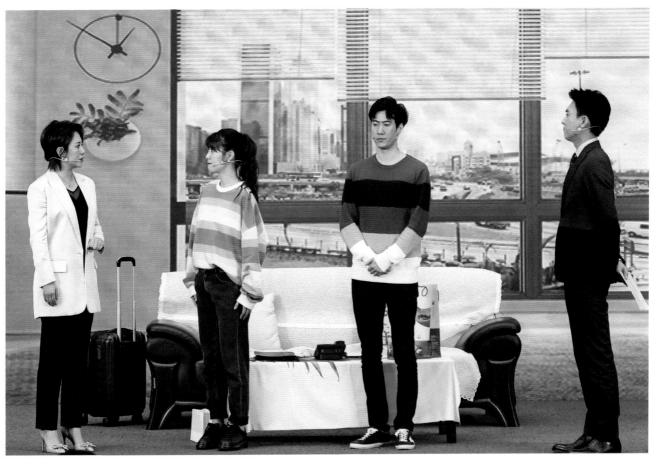

在2018年9月举行的第73届联合国大会防治结核病问题高级别会议上，彭丽媛应邀在会议开幕式上发表视频讲话。她说，正是由于中国政府和社会各界的关爱和重视，包括70万志愿者的热心参与，中国结核病防治工作近年来快速发展，广大患者正获得更加及时有效的诊断和治疗，结核病防治在一些地区正成为脱贫攻坚工作的一项重要内容，很多人因此重获新生。但人类在防治结核病方面仍面临严峻挑战，各国应携起手来，为终结结核病竭尽全力。

At the 73rd session of the United Nations General Assembly (UNGA) High-Level Meeting on Tuberculosis in September 2018, Madame PENG Liyuan was invited to give a video speech at the opening ceremony. She said that it is precisely because of the care and commitment of the Chinese government and the different sectors of the Chinese society, including the heart-warming participation of 700,000 volunteers, China has seen rapid progress on tuberculosis prevention and control in recent years. The large number of patients have been able to receive more timely and effective diagnosis and treatment. Tuberculosis prevention and control is becoming an important component of the tough battle of poverty alleviation in some regions. Many people have been able to get their life back. But mankind still faces serious challenges in the fight against tuberculosis. We as countries should join hands, Do your best to end tuberculosis.

我们相信公益的力量是可以传承的。无论是凛冬将至、前路漫漫、抑或风雨兼程，我们始终相信公益大使们将会用爱与行动温暖全社会，鼓舞人们在未来的岁月里勇敢地与结核病抗争，活出灿烂美好的人生！

We believe that the power of a good deed can be passed down. Despite any hardship or setback that lies ahead, even if the road is winding and bumpy, we always believe that our goodwill ambassadors could warm the society with love and action, encourage people to courageously fight tuberculosis in the years to come, and to live a wonderful and happy life!

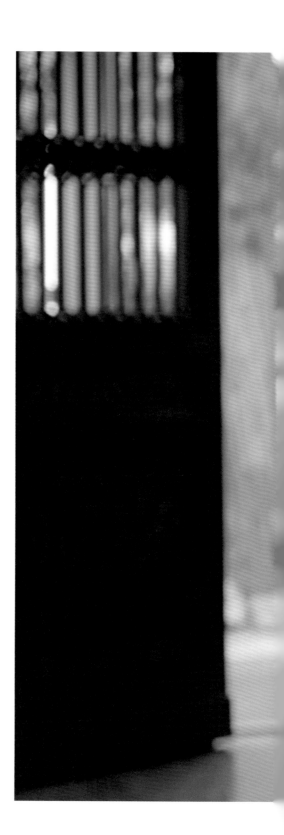

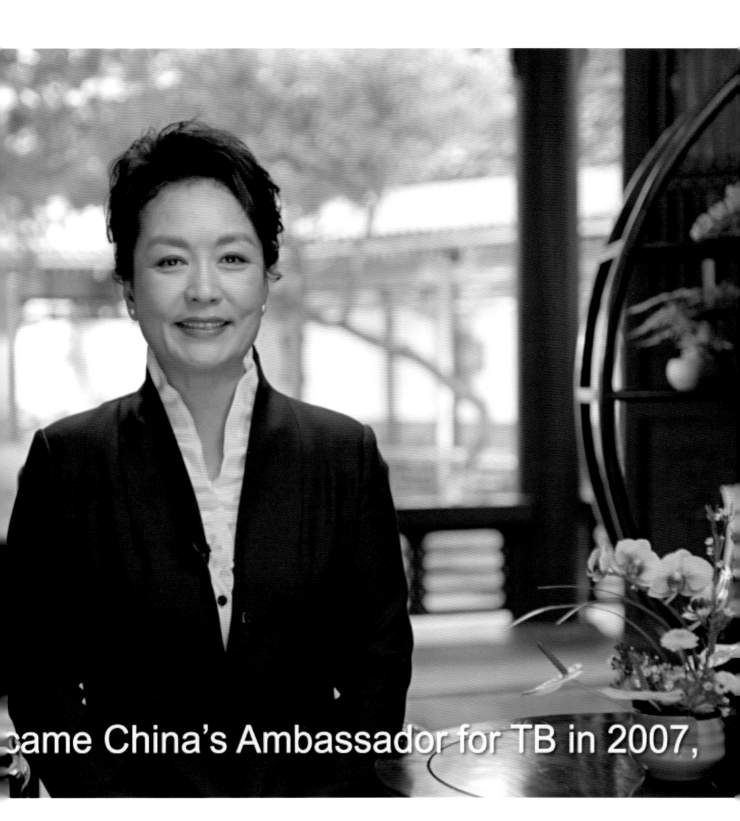

came China's Ambassador for TB in 2007,

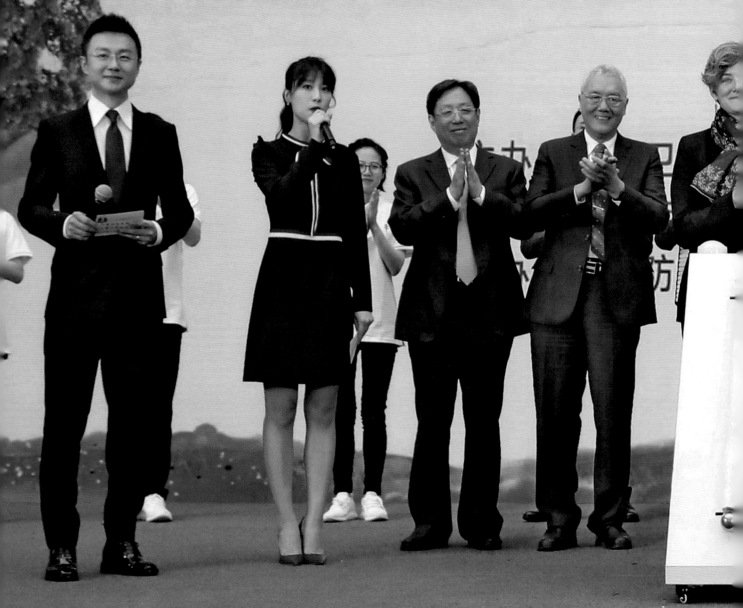

2019年 北京 2019, Beijing

编后记
Postscript

进入21世纪以来，虽然我国结核病防治工作取得了令人瞩目的成就，但是还面临着诸多问题与挑战，防治形势依然严峻。我国仍是全球30个结核病高负担国家之一，每年报告新发结核病患者近80万人，位居全球第3位；防治服务体系尚不完善，定点医疗机构诊治条件和设施设备严重滞后于防治工作需要，部分新型快速诊断技术应用尚不普及；患者医疗费用负担较重，部分患者自付医疗费用超过自身承受能力；一些防治难点有待突破，包括流动人口结核病、耐多药结核病、学校结核病等。在世界范围内，尚未研发出有效疫苗，缺乏新型药品及治疗方案。面临诸多挑战的同时，我们也有良好的机遇，2018年9月，联合国组织召开防治结核病问题高级别会议，发布了《关于防治结核病问题的政治宣言》，这将有力地推动世界卫生组织终止结核病流行目标的实现。中国将在习近平新时代中国特色社会主义思想和党的十九大精神指引下，认真落实全国卫生与健康大会的决策部署，为建设健康中国和全面建成小康社会作出积极贡献，最终实现终止结核病流行的目标。

Since the start of the 21st century, although China has achieved remarkable achievements in tuberculosis prevention and control, it still faces many problems and challenges. China is still one of the 30 countries with the highest burden of tuberculosis in the world. The number of notifications is nearly 800,000 per year, ranking the third in the world. The prevention and control service system is not perfect. The conditions for diagnosis and treatment at designated medical institutions and facilities and equipment are seriously behind the needs of prevention and control. Some new rapid diagnostic techniques are yet to be widely adopted; patients have to pay medical expenses than they can afford; some difficult and complex prevention and control challenges need to be addressed, including tuberculosis within the migrant population, multidrug-resistant tuberculosis, and tuberculosis at school. Worldwide, effective vaccines have not yet been developed, and new drugs and treatment options are lacking. While facing many challenges, we also have good opportunities. In September 2018, the United Nations organized a High-Level Meeting on Tuberculosis and released the Political Declaration on Tuberculosis Control, which will effectively advance the World Health Organization's goal towards ending tuberculosis. Under the guidance of General Secretary XI Jinping's thought on socialism with Chinese characteristics for a new era and the guiding principles of the 19th National Congress of the Communist Party of China, China will conscientiously implement decisions and deployment of the National Health Conference, and make positive contributions towards fully achieving the Healthy China targets and building a moderately prosperous society in an all-round way and ultimately attaining the goal of ending tuberculosis.

图书在版编目（CIP）数据

为了健康的呼吸：中国结核病防治纪实 / 中国疾病
预防控制中心等组织编写 . —北京：人民卫生出版社，
2021.2

ISBN 978-7-117-31295-0

Ⅰ. ①为… Ⅱ. ①中… Ⅲ. ①纪实文学 – 中国 – 当代

Ⅳ. ①I25

中国版本图书馆 CIP 数据核字（2021）第 035495 号

为了健康的呼吸——中国结核病防治纪实
Weile Jiankang de Huxi——Zhongguo Jiehebing Fangzhi Jishi

组织编写	中国疾病预防控制中心
	中国健康教育中心
	中国防痨协会
	中国性病艾滋病防治协会
出版发行	人民卫生出版社（中继线 010-59780011）
地　　址	北京市朝阳区潘家园南里 19 号
邮　　编	100021
印　　刷	北京雅昌艺术印刷有限公司
经　　销	新华书店
开　　本	889×1194　1/16　　印张：13.5　　插页：2
字　　数	427 千字
版　　次	2021 年 2 月第 1 版
印　　次	2021 年 9 月第 2 次印刷
标准书号	ISBN 978-7-117-31295-0
定　　价	298.00 元

E – mail　　pmph @ pmph.com

购书热线　　010-59787592　010-59787584　010-65264830

打击盗版举报电话：010-59787491　　E-mail：WQ @ pmph.com

质量问题联系电话：010-59787234　　E-mail：zhiliang @ pmph.com